Crystals for Beginners

Cleanse Your Soul and Be Happy Everyday

(A Complete Guide to Understand Energy and Healing Power of Crystals)

Richard Bagby

Published By **Ryan Princeton**

Richard Bagby

All Rights Reserved

Crystals for Beginners: Cleanse Your Soul and Be Happy Everyday (A Complete Guide to Understand Energy and Healing Power of Crystals)

ISBN 978-1-7780570-7-6

No part of this guidebook shall be reproduced in any form without permission in writing from the publisher except in the case of brief quotations embodied in critical articles or reviews.

Legal & Disclaimer

The information contained in this book is not designed to replace or take the place of any form of medicine or professional medical advice. The information in this book has been provided for educational & entertainment purposes only.

The information contained in this book has been compiled from sources deemed reliable, and it is accurate to the best of the Author's knowledge; however, the Author cannot guarantee its accuracy and validity and cannot be held liable for any errors or omissions. Changes are periodically made to this book. You must consult your doctor or get professional medical advice before using any of the suggested remedies, techniques, or information in this book.

Upon using the information contained in this book, you agree to hold harmless the Author from and against any damages, costs, and expenses, including any legal fees potentially resulting from the application of any of the information provided by this guide. This disclaimer applies to any damages or injury caused by the use and application, whether directly or indirectly, of any advice or information presented, whether for breach of contract, tort, negligence, personal injury, criminal intent, or under any other cause of action.

You agree to accept all risks of using the information presented inside this book. You need to consult a professional medical practitioner in order to ensure you are both able and healthy enough to participate in this program.

Table Of Contents

Chapter 1: The Power Of Crystals 1

Chapter 2: How To Choose The Right Crystals For Yourself 19

Chapter 3: How To Use Crystals To Balance Energy 31

Chapter 4: Maximizing The Power Of Crystals 39

Chapter 5: 10 Main Crystals 63

Chapter 6: Other Important Crystals To Realise 94

Chapter 7: What Crystals Can Do To Help Us In Life? 111

Chapter 8: How To Purify Crystals 119

Chapter 9: What Are Crystals? 127

Chapter 10: How To Apply Crystals The Right Manner: Strength And Notion 138

Chapter 11: The Power Strings And The Concept Of Vibration 146

Chapter 12: Benefits Of Crystal Treatment 159

Chapter 13: Creating The Best Crystals Grid 167

Chapter 14: History Of Crystal Healing . 175

Chapter 1: The Power Of Crystals

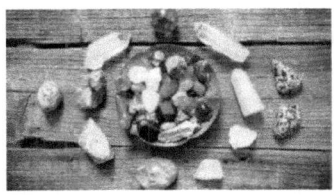

The fascinating trends of crystals had been used by mankind because of the reality life. Hematite and quartz had been used by the Ancient Greeks to hold off evil spirits and offer protection for the duration of war, at the identical time because the Ancient Egyptians wore stones like turquoise and lapis lazuli for adornment. Alchemists used crystals and natural mixtures to create potions inside the route of the Renaissance to useful aid in healing and illness prevention. Even these days, after centuries, these uncommon stones' electricity remains gift. What significance do they have got now, and how can we examine them to our everyday lives?

1.1 Power of Crystals and Modern World

Different stones have awesome consequences primarily based on the individuality of absolutely everyone. As a quit end result, our usage of them and our response to them are actually specific. The identical is actual of their blessings. Our strength is filtered thru crystals. They can consequently be applied to name forth now not simplest what we're looking for, which incorporates vitality, love, or self perception, but additionally to do away with that now not serves us. People can choose some crystals from a preference. They can continuously instinctively choose out the portions they require on the time. They do this to sell serenity or to rejuvenate existence. It's high-quality how properly this works at regaining a enjoy of power. It is also crucial to describe the stones' inclinations. It's important to explain what every shape of crystal does. One can installation a better bond with a crystal and with themselves once they have a radical data of the way each one abilities. The use of these lovely minerals dates all over again to historic Egypt, while it became believed that they is probably used to force out evil spirits. Crystal treatment has been done for some time to assist heal the frame holistically for pretty some troubles. These days, crystal remedy has shed its "hippy" photo and earned a much huge following from humans looking for to heal their frame certainly and make certain overall well-being. This is attributed to celebrities like Victoria Beckham, Ella Woodward, Madonna, and Katy Perry who are advocating the blessings. Some human beings receive as proper with that thru interacting with the frame's power go together with the waft, unique stones like rose quartz, amethyst, and jade can realign the energy channels which may be blockading the body's natural float of strength and assist the body therapy itself. Certain crystals and stones have been said to beneficial resource within the treatment of a tremendous form of situations, from intellectual fitness issues like strain and despair to digestive troubles. Crystal treatment can be practiced in lots of ways, collectively with the sporting of jewellery crafted from precious stones &

minerals, the location of crystals in a single's walking or snoozing surroundings, or the steering of a expert crystal therapist who is aware about which crystals may be used to decorate the seven chakras, or "power facilities," of the human frame. Each stone is said to have a very unique electromagnetic charge that emits recuperation vibrations, allowing it to break up strength blockages and get topics shifting over again.

1.2 The seven chakras

Given underneath is a brief evaluate of 7 chakras

First chakra

Stability, safety and our number one wishes are represented via using first chakra. It is assumed to assist us feel steady in addition to fearless.

Second chakra

Second chakra is center of creativity. Moreover, 2d chakra permits us in expressing ourselves.

Third chakra

Third chakra is a center of private strength.

Fourth chakra

The fourth chakra is the power factor. It unites the decrease chakras of consider and the higher chakras of spirit. Moreover, fourth chakra connects our frame, thoughts, feelings and spirit.

Fifth chakra

It is positioned within the neck. Moreover, it permits us to explicit verbally. It moreover fosters our potential to talk our highest truth.

Sixth chakra

It is positioned a number of the eyebrows. Sixth chakra is also called the "1/three eye." Moreover, sixth chakra represents our instinct middle.

Seventh Chakra

Sahaswara chakra, or "thousand-petal lotus," is located at the top of the pinnacle. This chakra represents spiritual enlightenment and a connection to each the self and others.

1.Three How to capitalize at the electricity of crystals with the help of Chakras

To invigorate, deliver, and balance the pores and pores and skin, one can also use extracts of treasured in addition to semi-precious stones and minerals. This is a completely specific revel in that can be used to enhance the restoration outcomes of crystals. In order to restore the thoughts and realign electricity factors in the frame, you can clearly combine a slight exfoliating frame treatment to clean similarly to tone the skin with a deep flowing rub down at the same time as the usage of a set of semi-precious stones whose chromatic tone relates with the seven special chakra factors at the body. After this treatment, the pores and skin is nourished, velvety clean, and has a mild shine to it. The reputation of crystals has improved presently. Many human beings employ them for an entire lot of purposes, which incorporates safety, recovery, and manifesting their desires. There are a few everyday crystals that you can assume to appearance on earrings, on exhibition, or in an strength employee's series, which includes amethyst, quartz, and jasper. But what approximately lesser knowns? Read on to discover about the lesser famous stones in the crystal nation whether you are organized to growth your data of gem stones or add a modern-day gem on your series.

1. Four Power of a few healing crystals

Growing numbers of humans now preserve in thoughts crystals to be especially powerful strength amplifiers. They are concept to include restoration energies that might beneficial useful resource in physical and emotional restoration, guard the man or woman from awful impacts, and result in suitable consequences like happiness, success, and loads. They took many centuries to form. Too few people make an effort to learn about all of the particular varieties of sacred stones. Today's market is flooded with newly discovered stones, masses of which have been lauded for his or her recovery houses. Some of these are particular versions of already-identified crystals that could have been misplaced in the course of in advance mining operations. These can also have effective recovery houses. Crystals have full-size meaning in plenty of cultures and perception structures. Incorporating crystals into one's material cupboard and home decor is extensively visible as a form of self-care. A handful of the crystals and their crucial blessings are mentioned proper right here.

1.4.1 Chiastolite

Listed below are the appearance, houses and capability benefits of chiastolite.

Properties and appearance

The mineral aluminum nesosilicate is the deliver of chiastolite. A particular black move may be seen walking via the brown stone. It moreover is going through the call Cross Stone. Native Americans often deliver this mineral with them in the end of ceremonies and rituals because of the reality they strongly be given as proper with within the protection it can offer. Additionally, chiastolite is concept to help stress, blood movement, and different problems, among others.

Potential benefits

This crystal might also additionally offer protection in opposition to unstable energies, facilitate non secular connection, enhance the immune gadget, help hormone manipulate, have a calming effect, growth emotional resilience, beautify highbrow sharpness, and foster internal serenity. Chiastolite is useful whilst you are at a crossroads to your life as it has a strong connection to the inspiration chakra. The frame's chakras are believed to be strength hubs which have an effect on your well being. It helps the cultivation of nice strength. It moreover helps in restoration charisma.

1.Four.2 Seraphinite

Listed beneath are the advent, houses and functionality blessings of seraphinite.

Properties and appearance

Crystals of seraphinite are a dark green shade with silvery streaks that capture and mirror slight. The Seraphim, the top notch order of angels, is historically pictured as sitting earlier than God's throne, and this gem is said to be their stone. Gems made from clinochlore, a magnesium-iron aluminum silicate, are extraordinarily unusual and handiest observed in Siberia's Lake Baikal area. Seraphinite is stated to incorporate a bargain power and hasten a person's increase on all stages of being.

Potential benefits

This crystal has the capacity to useful useful resource inside the release of limiting emotional patterns, beneficial resource in the restoration of the coronary coronary heart and lungs, stimulate the regeneration of cells, bring about emotions of happiness, harmony, and equilibrium, and help result in non violent resolutions to conflicts. As a forestall result of the nurturing energy radiated with the resource of this stone, the wearer is stimulated to help and have fun all styles of growth. Usually, it has some issue to do with the coronary coronary heart chakra, and it moreover offers energetic help for the lungs.

1.4. Three Tanzanite

Listed underneath are the advent, residences and potential blessings of tanzanite.

Properties and appearance

Blue zoisite, often known as tanzanite, is a calcium aluminum silicate gemstone. There is a large spectrum of blue tones to pick from, from completely see-through to very opaque.

Tanzanite is simplest located within the Merelani Hills in Tanzania, Eastern Africa, and because of this, it's miles every uncommon and expensive. As modern times, it has determined extremely good use in earrings due to the reality to the notion that sporting such an item might also additionally additionally boom one's meditative and psychic skills.

Potential advantages

Potential blessings of this crystal embody de-cluttering your surroundings, offering you with extra power, and decreasing your tension and worry. It may additionally moreover result in extra empathy, receive as authentic with, and introspection. Tanzanite is a stone of exchange that combines all aspects of connection and psychic electricity (transformation). Tanzanite is a stone that stimulates the 0.33 eye, crown, and throat chakras. This lets in deliver a lift to the hyperlink among our conscious and subconscious minds. It will make it much less difficult for you to tell the fact.

1.Four.4 Blue Siberian quartz

Listed underneath are the advent, residences and capability benefits of blue Siberian quartz.

Properties and look

Cobalt is used to create blue Siberian quartz, which has a colourful blue color, as the selection implies. It is artificial quartz superior in Russia. This precious gem is created by means of using fusing together fragments of herbal quartz which have been fractured and regrown with cobalt. Wearing this stone can, so the concept is going, decorate your telepathic and clairvoyant skills in addition on your psychic focus.

Potential benefits

The houses of this crystal consist of the enhancement of psychic vision and cosmic awareness, the promoting of tranquil feelings, and the encouragement of smooth verbal exchange. Those who address this stone document feeling a profound experience of calm. Since it retains a number of the quartz's houses, it could be "programmed" to enhance the restoration energy of other stones.

1.Four.Five Astrophyllite

Listed underneath are the advent, houses and ability blessings of astrophyllite.

Properties and appearance

This unusual crystal is typically formed like a spear and might variety in hue from a deep brown to a tremendous yellow. Potassium, titanium, iron, sodium, manganese, and silicates are applied in its manufacturing. It is also referred to as a Star Leaf. Some humans receive as actual with it is able to deliver them the strength to hold going when the going receives tough, assist them discover real happiness even in tough instances, and provide them path even as they will be at a crossroads.

Potential benefits

Hormone-balancing, ego-unfastened self-belief, psychic safety, faded regret and regret, greater sensitivity to touch, and eased launch of the beyond are all possible blessings of this crystal. Since astrophyllite heightens touch notion, it can be beneficial for individuals who make a living schooling rubdown or reflexology.

1.Four.6 Dumortierite

Listed beneath are the arrival, houses and capability blessings of dumortierite.

Properties and appearance

Dumortierite is a dense crystal that is often a deep violet or navy blue color. It is crafted from a very uncommon aluminum borate silicate. Some human beings trust that dumortierite's immoderate vibration can help them recall facts, growth their sensitivity to subtle cues, or maybe expand their psychic competencies.

Potential advantages

This stone has been used to address numerous ailments, together with headaches, nausea, shyness, vomiting, stress, phobias, or perhaps beyond-life trauma. It moreover permits human beings enlarge a healthy experience of self-love and self-worth. It is soothing and powerful at getting you to zero in on what topics maximum. Those who make their living in sectors in which strain and trauma are everyday partners will get the maximum from it. Keep a piece at your table to beneficial useful resource for your have a examine and bear in mind.

1.Four.7 Lepidocrocite

Listed under are the arrival, residences and ability benefits of lepidocrocite.

Properties and appearance

Lepidocrocite is an iron oxide hydroxide that paperwork in nature as an opaque, crusted crystal with red specks. The coronary coronary heart chakra is particularly stated to be aligned with and stimulated via using this gem. Emotional restoration and a higher connection to the heavenly power are other blessings.

Potential advantages

In addition to assisting with cell regeneration, liver feature, ADHD, hyperactivity, and melancholy, coronary coronary coronary heart and lung characteristic, restoration from abuse and trauma, and developing spiritual ties also are viable effects of running with this gem. While spotting your virtues, this stone dispels intellectual haze and allows you recognition. Learning to be more empathetic and lots a great deal less judgmental is one manner that Buddhism allows us triumph over the ego that holds us lower decrease back from granting others their entire diploma of employer. By bridging the gap some of the tangible and airy worlds, this stone allows its wearer update materialistic instincts with an unyielding love for the self and the surroundings.

Ethical stone sourcing is crucial

Before such as the crystal in your collection, affirm that it changed into mined responsibly. Overmining and forgeries may be avoided on this way. Earth is the deliver of many crystals, and the technique in their improvement can take masses of years. Since this is the case, they'll be scarce. Extremely uncommon crystals want to be bought with caution; when you have any doubts, you want to ask for proof of authenticity and probe the vendor approximately in which they sourced the crystals from. In current-day years, we've got seen a rise inside the style of stores that guarantee they satisfactory promote crystals from moral and environmentally accountable providers. Many specific styles of crystals exist; you may want to boom your collection to encompass a few you've got yet to peer.

Chapter 2: How To Choose The Right Crystals For Yourself

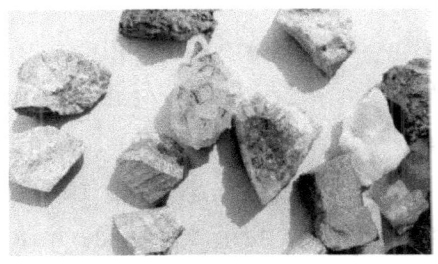

You have to do apprehend that finding a right crystal for addressing your issues is noticeably essential. Although that may be a difficult project, you can be triumphant if you have religion and herbal willpower. They can accomplish great topics on the same time as positioned with the motive of "I ask that this crystal bring and preserve a happy mood and maintain us constant, peaceful, happy, and energetically nicely." This is due to the truth that every crystal set below this purpose will start to function like a Wi-Fi hub, sending indicators at some stage in the whole house at that frequency and purpose. You need to exercise it earlier than you may determine what you are intuitively interested by on a given day. You ought to first determine what you want for the day, after which you need to reset your eyes and thoughts and allow yourself to be guided to what's required. To preserve us linked to the Earth and let you give up your anxieties over to the ground in place of allowing them to dance inner in and round your body and mind, you'll additionally want to find out some grounding stones, crystals which might be deeper in colour, together with Tiger's eye. You might be amazed to analyze that amethyst is a gem for maintaining an open mind and promoting precise sleep.

2.1 How do crystals have an effect on us?

Matter is sincerely empty place, constant with technological facts. And this clean location is complete of strength. Everything is crafted from electricity, and energy is everything. You, the seat you are in, the cellphone to your hand, & the crystals you are acquainted with and keen on. Every unmarried one folks has a awesome vibrational frequency that is just like some factor else inside the globe. While people with the lower vibrations are more likely to experience horrible feelings like jealousy, worry, rage, or worry, people with better vibrations emanate kindness, love, peace, and compassion. At any frequency, you, as a man or woman, have a very unstable vibration and are with out problems recommended through manner of the surroundings round you. As we engage with others, eat information, bypass approximately our each day lives, enjoy precise and terrible statistics, specific and lousy weather, fantastic and horrific reminiscences, and so on., it modifications always. On the very excellent hand, crystals have a totally steady electricity frequency. It is due to the truth that they may be composed of molecules which is probably prepared in a set, predictable, and nice geometric shape. And their specific stability is maintained with little attempt. In assessment to our very personal unstable, ever-transferring nature. So, why is it critical for a crystal to be robust? This is because of the truth that more potent strength is regular power. As a end end result, powerful power can have an effect on the energies in its vicinity. As a surrender result, we are capable of now recognize the amount to which crystals adjust our erratic (and so inclined) electricity.

2.2 Crystals & your chakras

Like people, every crystal emits its very private wonderful vibrational frequency. It is based upon on numerous factors, the most prominent of which being period, composition, and colour. So why does it virtually rely what colour a crystal is? What humans recognize as shade is honestly a spectrum of light frequencies. When in assessment to pink, for example, red is an extended way greater common. Indeed, the identical holds actual for our non-public our bodies. Due of its low vibrational frequency, the premise chakra (the lowest chakra) is depicted in pink on chakra diagrams. To the alternative, the very exceptional vibrational chakra, the crown, is associated with the coloration purple as it has the exceptional frequency. In maximum instances, the vibrational healthful amongst like colorings lets in you to choose out a stone that corresponds to the chakra you need to balance. Specifically, blue sapphires are useful for the throat chakra. Amber and yellow topaz crystals resonate with the sun plexus chakra. Nonetheless, rose quartz, which resonates with the inexperienced coronary coronary heart chakra, is an exception. But that is a terrific area to start although. If you do no longer understand which chakra to paintings on, allow your instinct guide you to the gem you may become loving except. Your instincts and physical makeup are constantly right.

2.2.1 Which crystals aligns with which chakra

According to Sanskrit traditions, the human frame includes seven chakras, or energetic points. These extend from the sacrum to the pinnacle of the top along the spinal column.

You need to furthermore be aware that each chakra relates to a positive body organ. The basis of all life electricity, usually called "Qi" or "prana," is the chakra device. Some crystals are also carried out to channel particular energies or dreams because of the truth they're related to precise chakras within the body or components of your lifestyles. Since the foundation chakra has the bottom vibrational frequency, its tendencies reflect this. It is commonly worried together along with your safety & bodily survival and is worried with the important additives of living. The more crucial emotions offer way to the richer, better vibrational feelings of pride, love, and creativity as you ascend the chakra device. The affects and activities in our lives might also motive an imbalance in our chakras. These imbalances may additionally need to occur as a intellectual infection, emotional illness, or bodily symptom. Crystals can assist in rebalancing any misalignment and bringing your energy centers once more to the frequencies they had been purported to vibrate at. Crystals be part of us to every our inner experience of ourselves and to our bodily body. It is well known that Chakra Heart Crystals have unique strength functions. Wherever your journey takes you, Chakra Heart Crystals help in bringing harmony and stability.

2.2.2 Restore your electricity through manner of aligning pink jasper with base chakra

Red jasper is notion to hold constant electricity, making it a mainly grounding crystal. As the "stone of staying energy," it fosters bodily electricity, stamina, attention, and remedy. Additionally, it alleviates fear and tension via improving feelings of safety and safety. When beginning a current employment or courting, keep a bit of red jasper close by.

2.2.Three You will have real fortune by using way of manner of aligning orange aventurine with sacral chakra

A stone signifying optimism and wealth is orange aventurine. It makes humans extra inspired. This stone additionally broadens your imaginative and prescient and brings success to you. Additionally, it's going to assist you to keep highbrow balance via lowering infection and aggression, bringing you again to peace, and selling emotional recuperation.

2.2.Four By aligning tiger's eye with the solar plexus chakra, you could rebuild yourself assurance

The tiger's eye is a image of bravery and self-guarantee. You might also see truely, stay targeted, and pass approximately your day peacefully with the aid of converting your angle. It moreover possesses a shielding exceptional and is historically carried to fend towards curses and horrible achievement. When you are worrying or afraid or whilst attending crucial meetings, deliver the stone with you so that you can also calm your nerves and revel in powerful and sturdy. Many oldsters are without a doubt insecure. Tiger's Eye is a effective self notion booster.

You ought to hold a chunk on your handbag whilst you want to counter the tough conditions. Additionally, it aids with highbrow attention and readability, which complements our sensation of manage and self-assurance.

2.2.Five When you align rose quartz with the coronary coronary heart chakra, you'll discover it to be very beneficial at strengthening your coronary coronary heart

Rose quartz is a adorable stone that could be a tender purple shade and represents unwavering love for ourselves, others, and the earth. It can assist us find out our soul mate, invite love, and heal heartbreak. It additionally acts as a reminder that the most vital love begins with self-love. Rose quartz is connected to stability, tranquilly, and peace. Keep rose quartz nearby to facilitate deep emotional recovery and to ease bodily stress. On a every day basis, all people want a touch warm temperature, and rose quartz in a slight red coloration is the precise stone for that. It is in reality suitable for luck and stylish love.

Your lives turn out to be greater "each day magic" and much less demanding as a surrender end end result. Keep a chunk to your pocket for whilst you desperately need a chunk convey.

2.2.6 If you're tormented by insomnia, then you could decorate your sleep through using the aggregate of amethyst and throat chakra

Amethyst is a crystal of protection and spiritual development. It improves mental clarity, opens up our instinct and emotions, and balances our feelings. Amethyst crystals are first-rate defensive stones for the home considering they each resist horrific electricity and draw remarkable energy. They also are helpful when you have insomnia, nightmares, or difficulties falling asleep due to the fact they let you lighten up. Amethyst works at the crown chakras, encouraging deeper sleep and mind relaxation in addition to enhancing reputation. As a end stop result, you may start and finish the day efficaciously. The crystal can be stored underneath the pillow, however it may also be positioned at the foot of the bed or at head top on a aspect table.

2.2.7 If you need to beautify your mind, then use lapis lazuli in aggregate with 0.33 eye chakra

For its functionality to stimulate the better thoughts and beautify cognition, lapis lazuli is fairly appeared. It promotes our thirst for expertise, truth, and facts and awakens the 1/3 eye, the place of inner vision and intuition. It additionally permits with analyzing and reminiscence. Lapis additionally evokes us to boom self-awareness and take rate of our life. Bring concord to a relationship or beautify communique by means of the use of wearing lapis lazuli.

2.2.Eight Clear quartz while aligned with crown chakra will can help you clean the thoughts

When finished to a sore region, clean quartz, a high-quality healing stone, is supposed to ease pain. Because it enables cognizance and consciousness whilst clearing the thoughts, this quartz is likewise visible as being useful at paintings. A clean quartz crystal is ideal to position on, supply, or use at some point of meditation because it opens the mind and coronary coronary heart. It is likewise useful to hold or have nearby if you experience uncertain or want to pay attention and word your way greater in reality because of its balancing and cleansing trends.

2.Three How to get the most out of crystals?

When they may be no longer left to do the entirety on their non-public, crystals carry out at their superb. Combine the crystal's natural power together with your very private targeted mind and dreams for maximum impact. It's a well-known reality that during which idea is going, electricity flows. So, growth your remarkable mind and intentions with the resource of using your crystals.

Chapter 3: How To Use Crystals To Balance Energy

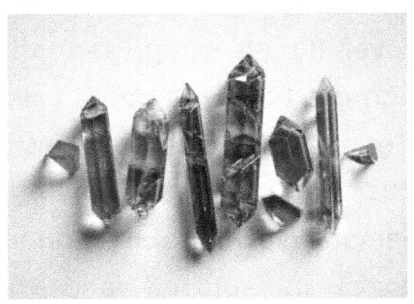

We have been looking for the sacred in nature for so long as we had been human beings. We have continuously been interested in crystals, rocks, and precious stones for numerous reasons, which include their aesthetic enchantment, the vibrations they produce, or a few issue more profound. Since we're creatures of the earth, it stands to reason that retaining onto part of it might deliver us solace and fortitude. If you start to hook up with crystals, then it will become a totally personal exercising. Anyone who has worked with or accumulated crystals will tell you that your very very personal reaction to a state-of-the-art crystal is the most critical hobby. Of course, you could choose crystals primarily based on the features you need to apply them for, however it's also important that you're feeling a connection with and a calling in the direction of a specific crystal. A crystal is most effective as effective because the effect it has on you personally; this connection will create the strength in yourself and inside the environment. In order to research greater approximately a crystal and determine whether or not it's miles suitable for you, many crystal companies will invite you to bodily have interaction with it. If this isn't always viable, however, examining crystals which might be available from numerous net retailers and seeing which ones you dedicate the maximum interest to can function an possibility. We are conscious that every crystal is specific to its owner, but we also are aware that many crystal kinds have the capability to generate and refine lots of energies and trends. In order to help you increase and balance the electricity you want on your settings, we can talk about the most famous crystal kinds and their meanings.

three.1 Energy stability and crystals

Crystals purge the frame of any negative electricity, which allows it hold stability. Due to their capabilities, which encourage healing, reduce strain, and useful resource in treating distinct commonplace problems, they also have satisfactory results on physical fitness. Since they bring about appropriate energies into our lives, many individuals hire them for spiritual functions. There are severa strategies to use crystals these days, together with wearing jewelry made from them, adding them into your beauty normal, and using them for meditation. The phrase crystal is also used frequently, whether or not or no longer it's in connection with skin care objects or style accessories. But now not every person is aware of the advantages the ones jewels can provide or how to excellent employ them. There is lots more than what the attention can see. Crystals as well as gem stones have unique benefits for our bodily, intellectual, and emotional properly-being. By putting in place a non secular connection among you and your self, crystals encourage self-love. With their gentle energy, moreover they assist in bringing your feelings into concord. The crystals beneficial resource in letting skip of horrible energies and preventing fatigue. The pores and skin, hair, and nails gain from them due to their nourishing inclinations. Crystals are mainly useful in improving consciousness and fostering each creativity and attention.

three.1.1 Agate can be used for accomplishing balance

Agates may be found in a huge kind of colorations and bureaucracy, but they'll be all useful for bringing balance. Many emotional imbalances, along with rage and terrible self esteem, may be resolved thru agates. Moreover, agates additionally resource in growing internal strength. Agate can often provide you extra electricity and power by boosting your self assurance and mind-set.

3.1.2 Amethyst may be very effective in removing stress and negativity even as boosting energy

Amethyst is super for promoting contentment, decreasing strain, and providing calm and rest. It silently offers us a lift in power and protection on the identical time as on foot to put off stress and negativity. When we allow ourselves to cognizance on our goals, amethyst can also be a exquisite useful resource for figuring out them.

3.1.Three You may be protected from threat with the aid of black tourmaline

A robust protector, tourmaline excels at driving away poor energy from our environment and minds. You can in reality hire black tourmaline due to its potential to characteristic a guard. Thus black tourmaline may be very powerful in shielding you from harm and negativity.

three.1.Four Energy is purified through crystal quartz

Crystal quartz is extraordinary in that it is able to talk with each one-of-a-type crystals and humans. It connects to each chakra in our frame, bringing internal peace closer to us. It ought to make our intentions clearer, purge our emotions, and energize us. The vibrations of the crystals nearby may be amplified with the resource of crystal quartz, making the ones crystals more powerful as properly.

3.1.Five Moonstone is beneficial for calming and balancing inflated egos

This stone gives a calming female air of secrecy, just like the moon. Moonstone can help you attain stability with yourself and exclusive humans thru calming, softening, or maybe taming effective egos.

three.1.6 Rose quartz aids in channeling love for oneself and others

Rose quartz crystal, that's red in color, is cautiously related to the coronary heart chakra and is excellent for attracting loving energy for ourselves, awesome humans, and the complete worldwide. When we want love the maximum, rose quartz can help us collect it for ourselves or open our hearts to offer it to others. This inflow of love can assist in clearing up minor annoyances and petty grudges, liberating us from negativity.

3.1.7 We experience enlightened with the useful resource of selenite

Selenite emits a terrific, natural vibrational strength which could remove darkness from entire space. This crystal is the epitome of purification and cleanliness, washing away staleness, negativity, and limitations. Selenite can uplift and enlighten us through the use of helping us in accomplishing a higher level of reputation.

three.1.Eight Turquoise permits in fostering honesty

Due to its blue color, turquoise has a relationship to the throat chakra, which governs speech. Turquoise can therefore promote honesty and openness, even inside our private minds. It works to hold your personal health at the leading fringe of your mind and is a effective promoter of health.

Chapter 4: Maximizing The Power Of Crystals

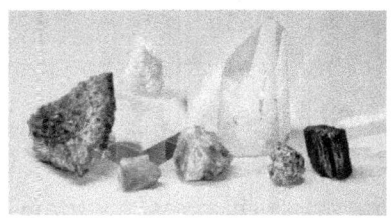

Crystals are a wonder for their innate splendor and healing powers. However, if you make use of crystals for additonal than really their mystical aesthetic, you have to wash them regularly to make sure that their frequencies remain natural, powerful, and easy. The healing functionality of stones may be maximized if you can find out a manner to apply them that works for you. To achieve fulfillment in crystal recovery, you need to understand the expertise of cleansing crystals. In the equal way that we need to clean our apparel after wearing them and dust our cabinets every so often, crystals require some religious maintenance to ensure that they stay powerful recuperation device. To hold a crystal in its maximum effective kingdom, it need to release a number of the more energetic facts it has saved via frequency and vibration. When you cleanse a crystal, you're basically wiping the slate clean and allowing your self to rewrite your lifestyles's tale with a glowing intention. It does no longer have an impact at the crystal's underlying energy resonance. It is notion that every type of crystal has its very non-public precise set of restoration powers. However, so as for us to align with them, their electricity fields need to be primed and organized to give & accumulate with out being inhibited thru undesired non secular muddle. Keeping your private recuperation crystals easy will repair and preserve their maximum natural recuperation capability. Unwashed crystals can also harbor a number of dangerous energy they've picked up on their travels. But once they had been purified, crystals can be programmed with our desires and used for his or her calming forms of strength. You can attempt out numerous strategies to cleanse crystals relying on the crystals you're managing and your private instinct. There are severa strategies for charging crystals to maximise their effectiveness. Because crystals generally tend to preserve onto the electricity that is directed to them, this power is fantastic on occasion useful. For instance, while you make use of a crystal for safety, the stone takes within the power it is meant to deflect. As a stop stop end result, periodically discharging the horrific electricity saved to your crystal is crucial. Like our our bodies need to recharge each night time time when we go to sleep, so does it. To get the most from your crystals' magical houses, here are a few simple techniques to cleanse them. Whether you want to rid your rose quartz of an everyday vibe or discern out a manner to purify selenite, you may discover the information you want right here.

4.1 Maximize the electricity of crystals via putting them below moonlight and daytime

One of the suitable and only tactics to cleanse crystals, in particular in case you are into astrology, is to go away them out inside the solar or moonlight. The whole moon is a effective section of the lunar cycle and a exceptional time to cleanse and recharge your precious crystals. Put the crystal at the ground out of doors at the night time time of a complete moon for it to soak up the moon's energy. You can use any flat, indoor window sill to enjoy the moonlight. As a cosmic cleanse, it'll rid your stones of any poor electricity and improve their incredible traits. The sun will assist your crystals, while the complete moon will take away any negativity or contamination they'll have accumulated. Put your first-rate foot in advance or some problem fits your dreams great. Your crystals will benefit in addition from an afternoon of sunbathing as from a night time time of moonlight bathing. The solar and moon have the energy to alter even the darkest & heaviest of vibes, so this technique is especially useful if you are attempting to parent out a manner to purify moldavite or black tourmaline, effective stones that may consume hundreds energy.

Benefits of charging your crystals with sunlight hours

Charging your crystals in the solar can be the quality desire for you if you need to price them with prosperity, love, and energy. The maximum applicable times to show the crystal to direct daytime are ultimately of the top notch morning and afternoon rays, but for incredible effects, leave it uncovered for as a minimum 12 hours. The strength that may be implemented to charge your stones is available in some unspecified time inside the future of various additives of the solar cycle. The wintry weather solstice widens the meditative place and lessens strain. The spring equinox promotes internal religious increase and boom in all spheres of existence. When choosing the way to fee your crystal, maintain in mind that some crystals will fade if exposed to the sun for a prolonged term. Amethyst, Sapphire, Aquamarine, Kunzite,

Aventurine, Fluorite, Beryl, Rose Quartz, and all gentle stones and minerals are examples of crystals a very good manner to vanish.

Benefits of charging your crystals with moonlight

The moon's electricity is remarkable for recharging your crystals. However, you must be familiar with the system and the moon, together with its levels, so one can gain this efficiently and in a manner that is awesome to you. The ascending moon brings wish, optimism, and new beginnings. The entire moon brings prosperity and love. Debts, negativity, as well as infection will all be removed via the descending moon.

four.2 Use Salt for maximizing the energy of crystals

Many humans use salt in non secular rites, which encompass bathing or growing a circle round themselves to protect themselves. Cleaning your crystals follows the identical policies. Partially bury your crystals in a dish of sea salt and set it aside. Then, go away them for the salt's cleansing consequences to take impact over the route of many hours or an entire night time time. Be conscious that moldavite, opal, & turquoise are the various stones that might be broken via prolonged exposure to salt. If you plan on using this approach, you want to make certain your crystals can manage being submerged in salt water. Stones, which encompass opal, calcite, and turquoise, are effortlessly scratched, so that you want to no longer use this method on them.

four.Three You can also use sound to cleanse and maximize the strength of crystals

This is why the sound of a gong or crystal growing a track bowl can be so reassuring and relaxing. The identical technique may be used to soothe your crystals' sensitive vibrations. Through the usage of sound waves, it's miles viable to launch blocked power and split energetic styles. Changing the frequency of your stones' energy with tuning forks, quartz bowls, chimes, or drums will help release any pent-up power. To reduce the horrible electricity emanating out of your crystals, take a look at with one in every of a type sounds and bear in mind your gut to inform you what works high-quality.

4.Four Water is also very beneficial for maximizing the strength of the crystals

Cleaning your crystals, the old fashioned manner with water will no longer handiest put off the accumulated dust on them but will even supply them a miles-wished strength enhance. A basin of water could possibly function a bathtub for the crystals. Natural water from the rivers, rain, or ocean is right, but water from the faucet will suffice in a pinch. Submerge the stones in water for at least 20 minutes and up to 2 hours. In order to similarly purify and reconstruct your frame, you can add a pinch of sea salt to the water if you so pick out. Stones additionally may be washed in a flow, river, or the sea. This is one of the simplest and maximum direct methods to easy your rose quartz, smooth quartz, or amethyst when you have been having trouble. Since most quartz is proof against water, that is the case. Each crystal in your stock requires individual studies to decide if it could efficaciously be wiped smooth in water. The -ite minerals (azurite, selenite, angelite, and so forth.) want to not be immersed in water. This serves as a robust guiding principle. Learn in case your crystals may be submerged in water to protect them from harm.

four.5 Cleanse and maximize the strength of crystals with smoke

Using smoke from an aromatherapy stick or a burning package deal of dry herbs is a honest way to release any terrible electricity that has become lodged on your crystals. To hold your crystals smooth and free of negative power, smoke them every day. It is crucial to discover ways to purify crystals with incense; the smoke from the incense can also cleanse your power location. This method works terrific in case you lease the smoke of herbs and vegetation recognized for his or her purifying homes. Light a package deal of dried rosemary, cedar, juniper, or resins like frankincense, pine, or myrrh to purge terrible energy from crystals and allow the smoke go along with the waft over and throughout the stones. In addition to ensuring that the cleansing system you purchase comes from top notch assets, you want moreover ensure that it efficiently cleans the area in query.

four.6 Crystals strength can be maximized phenomenally through burying them in soil

As earth's non-public superb creations, crystals can be cleansed and revitalized by way of reconnecting them with the planet's regenerative electricity. By permitting your crystals to make touch with the earth's inherent grounding power, you can help purge them of any negativity or impurities. Similarly, the ones polished stones are like buried treasure that has just been uncovered. Just make sure you bury them someplace steady. To put together the floor on your stone burial, scoop out a small quantity of the soil from the meant burial internet website on line and place it in a jar made from earthenware. Put the crystal deep down into the soil of the field. When you are accomplished, use the ultimate dirt to seal the tomb of the pot. Leave your crystal buried for now not much less than in keeping with week after you have marked it with a flag or other marker. It will permit your stone to take in greater of the earth's effective power.

four.7 You can also use wonderful crystals for maximizing the strength of your crystals

Even even though it might in all likelihood seem redundant, a few crystals have such powerful cleaning trends that they could even help different crystals launch blocked strength. The pretty excessive frequency emitted via the use of certain stones purifies the ones spherical them. Simply setting your crystals on those cleansing/charging stones for more than one hours will permit them to be charged and cleansed. Some examples of cleaning crystals that would be implemented on this fashion are selenite, kyanite, carnelian, and moldavite.

four.Eight Cleanse your crystals with visualizations for maximizing their power

Although using equipment to easy your crystals is amazing, it's also comforting to recognize that you without issues can also cleanse crystals with surely your mind. If you want to attempt using visualization to purify your crystals, begin via finding a relaxed region in which you could recognition and input a state of meditation. Holding the crystal interior your palms, visualize a super beam of white moderate emanating out of your 0.33 eye chakra, this is placed amongst your eyes on the brow. The mild ought to surround the crystal like a shield. Imagine that the mild has the capacity to transform something horrible into something notable. You have to observe your intuition in this situation. Continue doing this until you agree with your crystal has been nicely cleansed earlier than shifting without delay to the subsequent one.

4.Nine Soak crystals in moon water for maximizing their energy

Make your private moon water as an possibility moon-associated crystal charging desire. You can each submerge your crystals for approximately an hour on this moon water, or you may honestly pour the moon water on top of it. Again, satisfactory use stones that can resist getting moist.

four.10 Burning incense or herbs over crystals will help maximize their strength

Herbs and incense may be used to charge crystals. Pass your stones through the smoke of sage, sweet grass, Palo Santo, cedar, or incense crafted from sandalwood, lavender, or jasmine for 2 to three minutes to cleanse your stones.

four.Eleven Use your breath to fee the crystals and maximize their recuperation capacity

Crystals also can be cleared the usage of your breath. You must clean your mind of all outdoor mind earlier than you may clear a stone collectively at the side of your breath. Then, whilst although preserving the crystal in a single hand, exhale forcefully and wave your one in all a kind palm over the crystal unexpectedly.

4.12 You can maximize crystal strength through connecting the crystals to the spirit guides

You can be a part of the crystals with any spiritual courses or deities you figure with. You might take a second to ask the guides to connect with your crystals and your cause for them thru prayer or meditation.

4.Thirteen Brown rice may be used to cleanse crystals

Use brown rice to soundly clean your stones of negativity. To do this, location your stones right right into a bowl that has been full of dried brown rice. Give it a 24-hour damage. After you're performed, throw away the rice as it has absorbed all of the terrible power from your stones. Any stone can be effectively handled with this method, but protective stones like Black Obsidian, Black Tourmaline, Jet, Blue Kyanite, Fluorite, and Labradorite gain maximum.

4.14 Tips to preserve in mind

Charging crystals isn't a totally complex method. But if you are a amateur then you need to maintain in thoughts the subsequent elements:

• Find out if your crystals can withstand water or salt. Numerous quartz, amethyst, agate, moonstone, and citrine variations are examples of not unusual crystals that artwork nicely with water. Choose an alternate cleaning method in case you're unsure.

- Find out which detail the crystal belongs to. Look up each crystal's developments and discover in which they arrive from. For instance, malachite is installed to Earth, consequently it makes enjoy to bury it and charge it there.

- Clearing crystals as fast as you get them domestic from the store is often a remarkable idea due to the fact they'll bypass via severa fingers in advance than they arrive in yours. You can by no means ensure what form of power a person is keeping.

four.15 How do you software program program your crystals?

Crystals have inherent restoration houses, however it is able to be less complex to connect to the stone's energy when you have programmed it to remind you of your purpose in existence. The stone may be held in the hand at some point of meditation, positioned at the Third Eye (inside the center of the forehead), or maybe used whilst lying proper all the manner down to stimulate the Chakra similar to the desired final outcomes. Visualize your existence pressure merging with that of the crystals. Seek advice from the crystal regarding your gift try. Don't neglect approximately about to particular your gratitude to the stone.

4.Sixteen How to spark off your crystals?

In the occasion that your crystals have turn out to be useless or experience heavier than normal, electricity activation may be vital. Use your terms, breath, or music to impart some of your power to the stone. It's advocated which you take the crystal outdoor as nicely. Infusing the crystal with exquisite strength in a seaside or park also can have a large impact. To relocate your crystals, you can moreover rent an activation grid. It is viable to do that via surrounding the stone with active mirrors. A few of the most counseled crystals are apophyllite, carnelian, aventurine, rose quartz, easy quartz, kyanite, sodalite, ruby, and selenite. In order to simply faucet into the potential of your crystals, you have to take care to maintain them easy and charged always. Care on your crystals, and you deal with your very private existence, identification, and hobbies. Let's say you need to investigate greater approximately geodes and crystals or get commenced on your very very own journey with them. To beautify your private correct power, health, properly-being, love, and greater, an Energy Positioning Blueprint can guide you in designing a greater conducive workspace, domestic, or business agency.

four.17 How to cleanse clean quartz?

One of the most effective crystals to use for novices is plain quartz as it clearly magnifies electricity & is easy to narrate with. Additionally, cleaning it's miles definitely clean! Choose whichever of the aforementioned cleaning techniques you feel maximum cushty using in your precise quartz crystal.

4.18 How can selenite be cleansed?

Selenite does not require not unusual cleaning because of the reality it's miles a potently cleaning stone on its private. Smoke, sound healings, and cleaning visualizations are all alternatives in case you experience the want to purge an object. This is because of the porous nature of the piece, which necessitates keeping it faraway from moisture from the air, water, and salt.

four.19 How can amethyst be cleansed?

The calming, creative, and non secular traits of amethyst make it a wonderful crystal. A member of the quartz circle of relatives, this appropriate red gemstone, the majority of the cleansing techniques stated above are truly secure to hire. Try out many options to determine which feels the maximum effective.

4.20 How need to black tourmaline be cleansed?

Black tourmaline is one of the maximum powerful crystals which might be stated to be distinctly protective in opposition to any type of negativity. Regular cleaning is crucial due to the fact this stone absorbs a whole lot of power. Try purifying it with smoke, track, visualization, or via outcomes leaving it out in the sun's cleaning rays in desire to submerging it in water, that could damage the stone.

four.21 How can rose quartz be cleansed?

A rose quartz stone's coronary coronary coronary heart-recuperation & love-promoting vibrations can be extra with out problems attuned to on the equal time as it has been cleansed and purged of any stagnant electricity. Rose quartz may be nicely cleansed the use of almost any of the aforementioned techniques, collectively with soaking in salt or water, similar to clean quartz and amethyst. Choose something you found will art work the top notch.

4.22 How Can Moldavite Be cleansed?

In all threat, the extraterrestrial vibes emanating from moldavite are due to the truth that it's miles a powerful mineral usual through a meteorite. Because it cleanses strength, moldavite typically can be purified once in a while. However, in case you choice to head lower again in touch along side your cosmic roots, you can recharge it beneath a whole moon or depart it within the sun for a while. Just ensure you do not monitor it to any moisture or salt.

four.23 How can incense be used to cleanse crystals?

While smoke cleansing is one of the maximum not unusual strategies for clearing negative energy from crystals, it does not require any particular gear or a huge inventory of dried herbs to do. Clearing crystals is as clean as letting the smoke from some incense go together with the drift at some stage in the crystal as you attention on clearing away any negative electricity.

Part 2: Deepen your records of Crystals

Repeating, three-dimensional groupings of atoms, ions, or molecules are referred to as crystals. Any robust substance can crystallize, which include DNA. DNA crystals that can be visible with the naked eye had been these days made via chemists from Argonne National Laboratory, Purdue University, and New York University. The studies may be useful for growing nanoelectronics and prescription drugs. The oldest stated fragments of Earth's floor are zircon crystals from western Australia's Jack Hills, which date another time 4.Four billion years. It have become previously believed that the earth's center have become a single, 1,500-mile-great iron crystal. According to seismic investigations, the internal center can also genuinely be a set of tiny crystals in place of a unmarried sturdy. The bloodless, faraway limits of the sun gadget's icy comets were found to include tiny silicate crystals, which require great temperatures to shape. The required heat may also additionally moreover had been supplied through severe sun flares. The global's largest crystals, the ones gypsum formations can be so long as 36 ft and as massive as 6 feet, and might weigh as an lousy lot as fifty five masses, are determined in a limestone cavern 1,000 toes below the floor in Chihuahua, Mexico. A garnet weighing about 10 pounds turn out to be located in 1885 beneath 35th Street and Broadway, no longer some distance from in which the contemporary Macy's is positioned. Urban lore claims that it changed into located each by way of manner of a worker digging a sewer or for the duration of the development of a subway. The so-referred to as Subway Garnet became reportedly bought within a day for $100, or simply $2,300 in modern currency. Gemstones were once measured in clean gadgets. In Greek, a carat grow to be called a keration, this means that "carob bean" and modified into used as a reference for measuring tiny amounts. It weighs just like 2 hundred milligrams, or zero.007 ounce. It's said that Richard Burton boasted, "It has such lots of carats, it is almost a turnip," at the same time as he gave Elizabeth Taylor the heart-commonplace Taj-Mahal diamond. A "fancy vibrant purple" diamond without a doubt broke a international file on the identical time as a London jeweler paid $forty six million for it at an public sale. The largest gem diamond acknowledged to guy is—or alternatively, emerge as—the Cullinan diamond. When it have become positioned in South Africa in 1905, it weighed three,106 carats, or over a pound and a half of of, however it has considering been lessen into multiple hundred stones. The best Cullinan stones in the meanwhile are part of the British Regalia. One of the British royal scepters is ready with the maximum essential stone, a 530-carat behemoth. Salt, or sodium chloride crystals, are to be had to the relaxation oldsters. If all the water from the arena's oceans tired, all that is probably left might be four.5 million cubic miles of salt, or a dice measuring a hundred sixty five miles on each difficulty. Sugar is but some other commonplace crystal.

Chapter 5: 10 Main Crystals

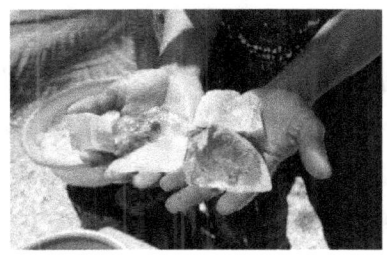

Listed beneath are 10 essential crystals and their healing homes.

5.1 Amethyst

Amethyst crystallizes as lengthy prismatic crystals internal geodes and unique cavities in rocks. These geodes rise up at the identical time as there are voids in an igneous rock, like lava. As the rock cools, the minerals in the water, gases, and volcanic material condense and crystallize. When those crystals harden, they remodel into amethyst. The stone's color can variety from a wealthy red to a reddish crimson or a very mild red that fades into lavender. Since at least the three hundred and sixty five days 2000, herbal amethyst has been prized for its splendor and applied in jewelry. On the Mohs scale, which measures the hardness of numerous gem stones, amethyst, and crimson quartz, are to be had at a strong seven. Gems crafted from amethyst are fine to be used in various earrings designs because of their resilience. Jewelry portions on the aspect of amethyst earrings, pendants, bracelets, and jewelry are very famous. Beads and bracelet bangles may be authentic from it as properly. As a end result of its hardness and sturdiness, the stone may be common right right right into a big type of office work, making it more malleable. Cabochons, bezels, and faceted stones are some of the most not unusual shapes. Natural amethyst of the first-class grade can be determined in big portions in Namibia, Australia, and the United States, in addition to in Siberia, Brazil, Namibia, Uruguay, and the Far East. The best amount of this valuable stone may be positioned in South America. The charge of an amethyst is based totally totally on numerous factors, collectively with its length and the depth of its coloration. Amethyst is a stone related to the 1/3 eye and crown chakras. The crimson to reddish-red tones of amethyst have lengthy been a sign of peace, purity, and calming power. The crystals constitute a proper away line to God and also the cleaning of one's soul. Amethyst is associated with beauty, peace, expertise, and keep in mind. This gem has spiritual undertones in step with many cultures. Amethyst is idea to provide restoration features that guard the wearer from harmful energies. Some people assume that the stone's enjoyable outcomes bring about non violent goals via raising our non secular recognition. The stone also helps communique some of the intellectual and spiritual geographical areas, which clears and calms the waking thoughts. It become as soon as believed that natural amethyst has the functionality to purge one's gadget of all pollutants. Ancient Greeks concept that wearing the stone avoided drunkenness and helped the wearer maintain a clean head. Amethyst stones had been applied in wine goblets to avoid drunkenness, and that they have been additionally located on ill human beings to attract out the contamination. Aside from its physical tendencies and benefits, amethyst furthermore has a chilled effect due to its crimson hue. It is supposed to assuage fury and tension, assist manipulate fears and anger, and burn up rage. Amethyst is also said to have the strength to dispel negativity and ease feelings of disappointment and grief. This gem's color is likewise related to awakening religious recognition, accepting intuitive electricity, and growing one's psychic talents.

five.2 Blue Tourmaline

Indicolite, a form of Indigolite, is every extraordinary call for blue tourmaline. The name alludes to the stone's stunningly deep blue color. It office work in solar sunglasses starting from moderate to darkish blue and is uncommon than distinct tourmaline crystals. Even some of them have a hint of turquoise. Typically, america, Kenya, Nigeria, Afghanistan, Sri Lanka, and Brazil are in which possible get blue tourmaline. Its coloration is severa and consists of a clean blue color among others. Compared to particular kinds of Tourmaline crystals, this one is uncommon. Due to the popularity of this particular mixture, blue and inexperienced tourmaline earrings is regularly advertised. When you have got a examine a blue tourmaline crystal, you'll experience calm because of the reality the photograph of tranquil blue waters will come to thoughts. It will purpose you to visualise yourself drifting gently on the ocean. This crystal will invite you to surrender manipulate of all of your mind and supply in to the solitude and calm of a tranquil, flowing stillness. It will inspire you to take part in a fantastic international of freedom and ascension to the moderate. As a stone of peace, blue tourmaline will provide a profound shape of meditation that lets in you to supply vintage wounds to the ground. It will inspire your get away out of your emotional attachments and the healing of your emotions. Additionally, it will will let you discover a deeper non secular bond and a greater reputation. Communication lucidity and honesty will enhance because of blue tourmaline. It will come up with the self warranty to specific your self brazenly and actual. Additionally, this stone will will let you open your thoughts, inspire you to certainly be given your self as you're, and inspire you to be more accepting of various people's versions and shortcomings. It will boom your feeling of obligation and foster a love for the truth. Additionally, it'll encourage you to stay a morally upright lifestyles and serve others. A lifestyles of concord and peace will be advocated, and blue tourmaline will inspire you to act with love and kindness. The throat and 1/3 eye chakras are related to blue tourmaline. It will decorate your clairaudience, clairvoyance, and clairsentience talents in addition to your connection to better stages of intuition. Your functionality to expect and speak with spirits may be unlocked. It's an extraordinary crystal, mainly for human beings intending to be medium or channel. When you get messages from distinctive nation-states, it will assist you procedure them and permit them to glide through your verbal verbal exchange. An exceptional crystal with a view to will let you absorb and remodel robust vibrations from the religious realm is blue tourmaline. It will allow verbal exchange with higher beings and assist you in channeling your restoration energies. By following your instincts and paying attention to the messages you acquire from the better geographical regions, Blue Tourmaline will assist you in attracting success and abundance. It will offer you with facts on specific financial conditions, allowing you to preserve with self warranty. It will assist you in overcoming beyond errors, setbacks, and disappointments. Additionally, it's going that will help you in connecting with those who can open doorways for you. Your efforts is probably rewarded via blue tourmaline, so that you can moreover can help you apprehend that you can benefit not anything in case you do not take a step in a selected route. In addition to supporting in the recovery of grief and sadness, blue tourmaline also can useful useful useful resource in letting pass of repressed emotions and antique recollections. You will open up and display all you have got been hiding from your sizeable one in all a kind. Although in the beginning it might seem intimidating, this could substantially alter the way your partnership works as a whole. It allows you heal from adolescence trauma, abuse, or damage mainly. You'll be capable to allow your right emotions and thoughts out in your expressions. Blue tourmaline has a manner of continuously ensuring which you and your accomplice can talk the truth and talk extra successfully due to the truth it's so carefully associated with the throat chakra.

five.Three Carnelian

Carnelian has the capability to captivate onlookers in the identical way that a beautiful sunset or the very preliminary burst of autumnal shade does. In addition to definitely being energizing and provoking, it stands for boundless enthusiasm, a welcoming surroundings, and eternal happiness.

Carnelian is a powerful and inspirational stone related to stamina, bravery, manage, energy, and concept. Humans have used the intense, wealthy hue of the Sunset Stone in a few unspecified time in the future of time as a deliver of motivation and protection. The historical Egyptians mentioned carnelians as "Sunset Stone" or "the putting solar" because of its orange colorings, which gave them a extra woman, docile, and receptive air. The stone is attached to the historic Egyptian goddess Isis because of her fertile and copious menstrual go together with the flow. However, even as the stone's colors are redder, redder-orange, and redder, it transforms into an active individual energy stone. Carnelian is frequently used to arouse love, desire, and passion because of the truth it's far belief to be useful within the ones areas. The orange coloration of this semi-valuable gemstone is derived from iron oxide. This shows that it's far quite easy to warmness-address, even by the use of really laying it out within the solar. The iron oxidizes whilst exposed to warm temperature, darkening the stone's pink colors. If you are within the market for a carnelian, this is something you have to apprehend. Your stone has probable been heated except stated in any other case. In Ancient Egypt, the Carnelian served many abilities, such as as a stone of fertility, an instigator of passion, and a source of braveness for the first warriors and fighters. Wizards used Carnelian in lands apart from Ancient Egypt. Using this powerful stone as a motive; they might set off exclusive stones. In addition to being a status symbol, many humans idea that with the aid of the use of honestly sporting the stone, they can be blanketed from harm. You can also locate the massive bulk of the location's orange Carnelian in India. Iron oxide and similar stones are vast in Brazil, Egypt, and Uruguay.

Carnelian stones have a long statistics of use as training aids, with claims of achievement in enhancing coordination and balancing strength ranges in some unspecified time inside the destiny of workout. Carnelian has been verified to boom muscular stimulation, bearing in thoughts higher oxygen distribution within the course of the frame. The warmth stone makes you experience "looser" and "freer" because it relaxes traumatic muscle groups. In addition to its distinct feasible benefits, this unusual gem also can moreover growth fertility and stimulate desire inside the mattress room. If you have got troubles in the bed room, try the use of Carnelian for help. Carnelian supports the Root Chakra, which in flip lets in the alternative three lower chakras it affects. Having a healthful 1/three eye chakra is vital for retaining equilibrium and stability. Carnelian is a crystal recovery stone that stimulates the appetite and lifts one out of a funk. It is also related to the sacral chakra. Near the end of this dialogue, we gather the Solar Plexus Chakra, which governs our experience of self, ego, and character. The energy of will that the Carnelian instills in us will see us thru any issues. Legend has it that wearing a carnelian stone can draw prosperity and genuine fortune to its wearer. Numerous people have found achievement through the usage of the use of this stone on every occasion they were in a pinch. Carnelian is a crystal of ambition, endurance, and pressure, and it is believed that those trends will defend the wearer from the slow energies of green coworkers. The stone's purported therapeutic effects can rationalize Carnelian's full-size attraction.

5. Four Citrine

Citrine belongs to the quartz mineral family. It may be any coloration of amber, from mild yellow to colourful sun shades of amber, and has its hue because of the fact iron is present in the quartz crystals. Citrine often has a hexagonal crystal shape and looks hazy or smoky in its natural us of a. Citrine's which means that is targeted on abundance, pride, and strength. Citrine is a stone of daytime that embodies summer time. You can not help but fall head over heels for the right away uplifting sentiments that sunny Citrine brings to the desk. It has the brightness of the noon sun, the color of lemons from the Amalfi Coast, and a touch of antique Hollywood glamour. This stone is colorful and energetic and is truely a completely particular shape of quartz that is usually yellow in color. Citrine comes from Scotland's highlands, Spain's flamenco regions, Madagascar's tropics, Russia's opulent and wealthy territories, and Brazil's lush inexperienced rainforests. Maybe it gets its terrific strength from the ones some distance off places, or perhaps it is actually Mother Nature's way of training us that when existence brings you lemons... Citrine crystal's golden shine changed into cherished as a wonderful decorative jewel as early as 3 hundred BC. Citrine changed proper into a famous gemstone utilized by historical Roman and Greek jewelers to decorate earrings worn on key fingers. Citrine maintained its repute as a valued gem regardless of the passage of time. Citrine end up a gemstone that Queen Victoria moreover cherished and wore in her seventeenth-century garb to create a declaration. Citrine have end up an iconic part of artwork deco fashion in some time, in a few unspecified time inside the destiny of the ultra-modern length of the Hollywood royalty, thanks to celebrities which encompass Greta Garbo who wore it at the pink carpet. The call "citrine" comes from the Latin word for lemon, and we recognize it for its candy and astringent energy. Beyond its aesthetic enchantment, citrine has loads of benefits that you have to recollect incorporating into your life. Citrine is like a summer season holiday on your soul. It can repair need, inject smooth power, and soothe strained nerves. Come with me as I discover the energizing and recuperation homes of the citrine stone. Citrine's yellow kiss will dispel gloomy feelings. This vibrant stone has a right away effect at the health and richness of your frame, mind, and soul and is usually equipped to supply positivity and splendor to the desk. You can generally rely upon natural citrine to take those difficult moments in hand and transform them into a few component superb because of the fact it is so blessed and fantastic that it can not hold onto bad strength. Here are some techniques that citrine is a superb investment for your nicely-being. Citrine does wonders for producing upbeat moods and warming the bodily body, much like status inside the gentle warmth of daytime. Citrine might truely be the stone if nutrition D had been a gemstone. You can also moreover kiss slow energies adieu whilst you consist of citrine into your existence. Citrine is a powerful power booster and may be a notable present for individuals who war with persistent fatigue or different health problems that drain your non-public reserves. Citrine is a stone to help you rise up through way of your bootstraps without knocking you off stability, despite the fact that it offers you energy. Citrine promotes healthy thyroid feature, a legitimate digestive gadget, progressed blood flow, and the suppression of allergic reactions and other pores and pores and skin irritations of a huge range. People who experience menstrual ache or a cycle that looks out of balance might also admire the soothing citrine houses, which can also be implemented to cope with nausea. It ought to come as no surprise that Citrine's pleased disposition is focused on effective strength, excitement, and preserving one's enjoy of self esteem. If you ever begin to enjoy like you've got out of place manage, Citrine may be there to inspire you to simply get it once more with a grin. It aids in clearing your thoughts, letting move of awful feelings like anger and resentment, and taking cleansing deep breaths that will help you remove mixed emotions like sadness and negative inclinations. Citrine instructs you to allow pass of everything that not makes you experience as notwithstanding the truth which you are being sopping moist in sunlight hours. Citrine's restoration strength assist you to overcome your fears with the aid of using reminding you that you are on pinnacle of things of your very own nicely-being and which you cannot fail. You can get entry to the ones abilties of manifestation while you revel in the go along with the go with the flow of pure optimism. You proper away sense like everything is viable even as Citrine is to your side, and it's far! You'll sense a stunning surge of self guarantee and be capable of go with the present day-day-day of existence in desire to fighting in opposition to it. It will enhance your resilience and teach you a manner to take positive complaint in stride. Citrine is a first-rate gemstone for individuals who actually enjoy the selection to ignite their modern coronary coronary heart as it emits a glow of innovative electricity. When you're moving beforehand with this excessive super wondering, it welcomes a enjoy of favor and flexibility, and you're unexpectedly capable of draw topics with a view to deliver you splendid pride yet again into your existence. People who put on this energetic and sunny stone are more likely to draw outstanding companions, wholesome relationships, and magical mentors.

five.Five Clear Quartz

A obvious, colorless mineral composed of silicon and oxygen is referred to as clean quartz. Clear quartz is beneficial in feng shui for reinforcing the effect of different crystals. Other benefits of clean quartz embody its capability to purify electricity and useful resource manifestation. A sturdy crystal with a recuperation and amplifying energy is plain quartz. All chakras reply pleasant to smooth quartz, which moreover may be carried out to cleanse the bodily and energetic our our our bodies. Increasing intellectual clarity is one of the benefits of easy quartz. It's implemented in restorative art work and meditation and can beneficial resource with emotional stability. It's often used for manifestation and can useful aid in bringing a choice into sharper recognition. It also may be useful in comprehending oneself, seeing topics from a unique angle, and seeing the reality of a situation. By exposing apparent quartz to moonlight or soaking it in water, you can clean and rate it. You can positioned on smooth quartz rings or convey a bit of it on your pocket or handbag.

5.6 Turquoise

Popular turquoise gemstone has lengthy been valued in a whole lot of cultures. It is one of the birthstones associated with December and is taken into consideration to offer pinnacle fortune, calm, and protection. Beyond the cultured value of the blue colour they provide, turquoise stones have masses of symbolic implications. Its strength is non violent, soothing, and defensive, making it beneficial for lots of feng shui programs.

Spiritual this means that of turquoise

If you could describe the turquoise's importance in a religious context, what could you are saying it's far? The stone offers a chilled, grounding power that makes it an super meditation useful resource or stone to use even as you sense beaten. It is stated to help you connect to the spiritual worldwide and to attach heaven and earth. In addition to being useful for protection and purification, turquoise allow you to enjoy extra related for your intuition.

Benefits and uses

The advantages of keeping turquoise stones in your private home are numerous. Turquoise has a sturdy connection to the throat chakra and aids in improving communique and expression. It is extensively employed within the remedy of illnesses further to balancing all of the chakras. Turquoise also can assist you triumph over toxic behaviors and enhance your functionality to love and forgive. You enjoy calmer and further snug because of its powerful emotional balancing results. Turquoise stones don't have any terrible outcomes.

Make your meditation area greater colourful with turquoise

Turquoise is the perfect stone for meditation since it balances feelings. It not excellent has a relaxing exquisite, however it may moreover help you in keeping you grounded whilst wearing out spiritual practices. Place a piece of turquoise within the part of the house wherein you need to meditate, and make a dependancy of connecting with the stone as you begin every day.

Activate your new beginnings region

One of the quantities of the feng shui bagua map related to the timber element is the New Beginnings location, or Zhen in Chinese. If you need help in beginning a today's project, you will likely need to spark off this vicinity. One method to activate this vicinity is to area blue and inexperienced stones there, like turquoise. Since letting bypass of antique styles is often important whilst starting some aspect new, turquoise's strength to dispel negativity and barriers may be mainly useful in this regard.

Bring calming strength into the bed room

The vicinity of your house in that you want to experience the calm and peaceful is your mattress room. It's important to have a place in which you can unwind, particularly in case you work from home or when you have younger youngsters or awesome family individuals who often want your interest. If your intention is to advantage from its electricity, positioned a cute, place a dish with a few turquoise stones subsequent for your bed. You can also additionally placed a tiny turquoise stone underneath the pillow to aid in a peaceful night time's sleep.

Activate your home workplace

According to feng shui, particular regions in your own home correspond to important components of your lifestyles, and the place of job is associated with your expert existence. Turquoise can be a useful addition to a domestic workplace because of its calming and grounding energy, which can help you live focused. Having turquoise within the home administrative center need to assist you deliver the ones developments on your artwork due to its functionality to improve communique and creativity.

5.7 Smoky Quartz

This powerful stone is darkish and mysterious. Moreover, this stone moreover has severa makes use of and medicinal advantages. This stone is for you when you have problem letting pass of antique conduct, beliefs, emotions, and concept patterns. In order that will help you ground into the earth, natural slight strength out from crown chakra is concept to be channeled down to the bottom chakra.

What is smoky quartz?

Crystalline quartz is available in diverse sunglasses, which incorporates smoky quartz. They may be a few aspect from a light yellow-brown to a darkish brown. Moreover, because of its colour, it could also be flawed for a black gemstone. The presence of radioactive minerals and special close by natural property of radiation gives this adorable shape of quartz its coloration. Irradiation is each unique technique that may be used to artificially produce the shade.

Benefits and healing homes of smoky quartz

Smoky quartz is an wonderful stone for grounding, as has already been referred to. Smoky quartz is known to cleanse horrific electricity, purify the frame and electricity area of decrease vibrations, guard the body from radiation, and treatment digestive troubles. These advantages are similarly to the numerous different restoration blessings of the quartz circle of relatives.

What chakra is smoky quartz actual for?

The root chakra is concept to benefit from smoky quartz. The chakra at the tailbone is called the idea chakra, controls emotions of balance, safety, and equilibrium.

How is smoky quartz used?

It can be worn for your frame as rings like necklaces or jewelry. Bringing this stone into your private home and place of work is every other powerful method to apply it. They'll bring all their soothing and uplifting functions into your room similarly to performing as one-of-a-kind and excellent decorations.

What is the first-class location for smoky quartz?

To take care of your root chakra, vicinity smoky quartz crystals at the bottom of the spine. Additionally, you could rent this crystal to stability the sun plexus chakra, that is positioned above your stomach.

five.Eight Rose Quartz

Rose quartz symbolizes compassion and love. The coronary coronary heart chakra communicates with the throat chakra. It communicates numerous kinds of self-care and compassion. It isn't always any mystery that rose quartz is a photograph of unrequited love. The rose quartz stone is established to the heart and throat chakras. Rose quartz lightly addresses all forms of love, from strengthening relationships with partners and pals to bringing sweeter undertones of self-care into your non-public lifestyles. Rose quartz is to be had in sun shades that beautify the romance thoroughly. Some Rose Quartz crystals have the color of a ultra-cutting-edge dawn, at the same time as others have a almost violet coloration. The cause of rose quartz is to energetically and tenderly unite your fragile coronary coronary heart with real and loving compassion.

Rose quartz physical healing houses

It complements coronary coronary coronary heart health and lets in to promote skip. Pregnancy can benefit from it as nicely. Rose Quartz not only has wonderful physical restoration talents however additionally works wonders for soulful recuperation. Rose Quartz can help to save you thrombosis and coronary heart assaults, beautify the circulate device, and make certain that your coronary heart muscle tissues are as clean and effective as viable. All the above referred to dispositions of rose quartz are consistent with its issue of being a coronary heart healer.

Mental & emotional recovery houses

It promotes emotional wound recovery. It encourages more kindness and care. For those who yearn for extra love in their lifestyles, rose quartz is often applied as a calling card.

Metaphysical homes

It fosters deep connection and attunes to goddess strength.

The exceptional manner for the usage of Rose quartz

It may be efficiently used on your splendor exercise workouts. The best use for it is as jewelry. To ensure that the heartstrings are gambling loud and clean notes, the Heart Stone have to continuously be nearby.

Office & Home

The mattress room is a inclined region wherein you may trap romantic thoughts, so it is endorsed that the Rose Quartz be organized on a particular altar there. Place the crystal outdoor the mattress room inside the center of the house to welcome visitors with love and super vibes.

5.Nine Fluorite

Fluorite is the proper crystal for each person coping with burnout, adversity, or pessimistic concept patterns due to its reputation for transmuting terrible electricity into right electricity. Fluorite earrings can boom your energy and beautify your air of mystery. Fluorite can enhance the immune device, sell highbrow readability, loose up blocked power, and help with physical cleansing. Fluorite can growth hobby, assist you hold in thoughts vital data, and enhance your significant mental talents. Fluorite may be nicely located sooner or later of your property to provide a robust Feng Shui harmonic effect.

Fluorite uses & chakras

Fluorite is a completely super stone that is available in almost all the solar shades of the rainbow, shimmering in hundreds of colours from easy to attractive pink tones and moderate blue sun sunglasses. Fluorite is frequently beneficial for balancing and harmonizing religious electricity. There are various colorations of fluorite and each has precise traits, including the following:

Green Fluorite

It allows to increase get entry to to intuition. To ground or soak up greater power, and to cleanse and regenerate the chakras, use inexperienced fluorite.

Blue Fluorite

It allows to prompt the Third Eye Chakra. This assists in boosting religious awakening and permitting unobstructed communication some of the material and spiritual worlds. Blue Fluorite helps orderly conversation and non violent, serene energy at the same time as used with the Throat Chakra.

Purple Fluorite

It stimulates the Third Eye Chakra and offer psychic intuitions a dose of purpose.

Yellow Fluorite

It allows to make instinct clearer and fosters innovation. It works wonders as a detox stone.

Clear Fluorite

For blending personal and religious forces, the Crown Chakra is the exceptional area to rent this.

Clear Fluorite lets you see the restrictions preventing your religious development and aligns all of the chakras.

Rainbow Fluorite

All the chakras may be cleansed way to the mix of tendencies that this fluorite famous.

Fluorite for clarity

For all people who desires a similarly growth of clarity in their existence, fluorite is the appropriate crystal. Fluorite can help through grounding you on your fact, cleansing your chakras, and purifying your charisma.

five.10 Hematite

Hematite is well-known for being a grounding stone with protecting homes. It is famend for being completely black and having a adorable steel shine. However, because of the excessive iron content cloth fabric inside the stone, it's far really blood purple in color. This crystal is a very strong and lengthy-lasting stone. The stone has a robust and strong shape. It may be visible most often in Brazil and South Africa. It is likewise present, even though, inside the Swiss Alps and on the Canadian borders of Lake Superior. Hematite is a crystal. This crystal is made from iron oxide and is an vital iron ore. Because of the iron recognition and the accompanying shine, the stone often appears to be steel. For this stone, black is the maximum everyday color. But it moreover is to be had in reddish-brown and brown. It is also available in silver and gray shades.

Chapter 6: Other Important Crystals To Realise

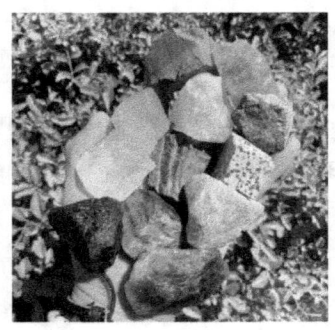

There are numerous special crystals with recuperation qualities. Now we are able to speak about diverse residences and recovery capability of some of the most important crystals.

6.1 Agate

Body, thoughts, and spirit can be restored to harmony with the usage of agate. It stabilizes the air of mystery and purges negativity. Agate improves highbrow average overall performance by improving focus, perception, and analytical capabilities.

6.2 Amazonite

Amazonite has long been believed to have a calming effect at the worried tool. Since the worried machine controls our emotions to a great quantity, it's miles believed that this stone can ease tension and foster romantic feelings. This stone is generally endorsed to be worn as a necklace across the neck, in which it is able to be held close to the heart and throat.

6.Three Amber

By collecting terrible electricity and generating fine, calming energy, Amber is said to calm nerves and revitalize the temper like a highbrow sunny day. Since amber is to be had in a rainbow of sunglasses, it is regularly used along side the colours associated with the seven chakras to help open and cleanse them.

6.4 Ametrine

It is stated that ametrine, the "stone of connection and balance," can reduce stress, result in a rustic of tranquility, spark innovative concept, and keep a healthful equilibrium amongst self guarantee and self-doubt. Since amethyst and citrine are every taken into consideration to be detoxifiers, it's far believed that ametrine presents a multiplicative effect in this location.

6.Five Apache tears

Apache Tears are a remarkable stone for repelling awful affects. The ideal stone for balancing one's strength vicinity is an Apache Tear as it absorbs negativity and shields the electricity frame from unwanted vibrations, energies, and entities.

6.6 Apatite

The gemstone is stated to lessen urge for meals at the identical time as enhancing comprehension, creativity, and analyzing (hunger). Apatite is said to beautify beauty, intelligence, and unconditional love. It is likewise said to growth intellectual clarity.

6.7 Aquamarine

Aquamarine, moreover known as the "breath stone," is extensively appeared for its beneficial consequences at the respiratory gadget. There are claims that it could moreover address a variety of allergies, bronchitis, and colds.

6.Eight Aventurine

Aventurine is famend for reducing anxiety associated with professional usual overall overall performance and promoting compassion, highbrow readability, and creativity. Aventurine stones are regarded to enhance the disturbing device even as moreover encouraging the thymus gland's successful function on a greater bodily level.

6.Nine Calcite

Compared to exclusive stones, calcite has the greatest packages. It is hired in loads of merchandise, collectively with paint, pigment, agricultural soil treatment, pharmaceuticals, acid neutralizer inside the chemical region, and manufacturing materials (within the form of marble and limestone).

6.10 Chalcedony

Self-doubt can be eased and internal peace may be attained through carrying chalcedony. It is concept that blue chalcedony encourages the client to accumulate peace with the resource of relaxing and centering the emotional energy. Healing: Individuals who have a unethical to end up worrying with out issues advantage maximum from using this gem.

6.Eleven Danburite

Crystals made from danburite have a cute, pure vibration this is very non secular. They are stones that have healing houses and a especially uplifting electricity. This stone's various shades characteristic first-rate catalysts for awakening and religious improvement. They are quite powerful for meditation.

6.12 Emerald

Emerald is a stone that promotes power. The coronary coronary heart chakra is opened, and the emotions are calmed. It gives motivation, harmony, knowledge, and staying power. It is supposed to permit the wearer to each supply and obtain unconditional love, sooner or later fostering friendship, serenity, harmony, and own family pride.

6. Thirteen Epitode

It lets in us to release different "heavy" emotions like grief, rage and tiredness. Epidote allows us preserve in mind that lifestyles is tremendous and that we each have particular obligations. It additionally permits us to soak up hard duties and remedy them with willpower and professionally. Epidote demanding situations us to be greater honest with ourselves while going via hard situations.

6.14 Fuchsite

Other crystals' power is prolonged and transferred extra effectively via fuchsite. By redirecting electricity into tremendous channels, it receives rid of obstructions delivered on through surplus electricity. Fuchsite improves musculoskeletal flexibility and stabilizes the area of the spinal column.

6.15 Garnet

Garnet cleanses the blood, keeps coronary heart fitness, and activates and balances the Root Chakra. Numerous advantages of garnets are to be had. It strengthens the spleen and lungs and heals spinal wire harm. Additionally, it reduces unhappiness, and in step with legend, the garnet stone shields the customer from poison.

6.Sixteen Howlite

Howlite is a completely emotional stone, however it additionally does plenty to promote bodily nicely-being. The bone-colored stone can beneficial resource in maintaining the frame's calcium levels in phrases of bodily properly being. You may also furthermore start strengthening your teeth and skeleton with this stone, and you can moreover begin growing extended, thick hair with it.

6.17 Jade

Jade, that's related to the coronary heart chakra, is robust in treating blood waft problems further to stress and tension. It is called the stone of affection, energy, and greatness and is set up to the coronary heart chakra and the Virgo zodiac signal.

6.18 Jasper

The only gemstone for lowering stress is jasper. It is stated be the "very excellent nurturer" and is stated to useful beneficial aid in calming down and mission serenity. It shields your electricity thru soaking up the toxicity, making it a useful tool to have reachable all through hard instances.

6.19 Kyanite

The robust stone kyanite has a tremendous form of beneficial makes use of. It offers a calming, centering vibration that may be used to get right of entry to meditation states as well as to stability emotions. The 1/three eye chakra is opened, and we are capable of use it to recollect dreams and hook up with our intuitive abilties.

6.20 Labrodite

Labradorite, a spiritually energizing stone, is stated to be of unique use to humans who have a dependancy of overworking themselves. In addition to assisting you experience greater energized, it additionally encourages your frame and soul to heal themselves. The metaphysical community considers labradorite to be one of the best defensive stones. The gem offers a protecting barrier for one's air of secrecy. It has furthermore been recommended that labradorite can help us sense an awful lot much less down in the dumps.

6.21 Lapis Lazuli

There are severa fitness benefits of lapis lazuli. It improves blood flow into, lowers blood pressure, cleanses the blood, and lessens any contamination the device may be experiencing. It is likewise said to deal with issues with the thyroid, throat, and melancholy, in addition to insomnia. It benefits the neurological gadget and the respiration system.

6.22 Larimar

Larimar is perception to have non secular, emotional, highbrow, and bodily recovery homes. An boom in hobby is felt within the thymus, 1/3 eye, throat, and crown chakras., promoting both inner facts and outward manifestation. It represents calmness and readability and exudes a loving and recuperation strength.

6.23 Lodestone

It will artwork with you to draw some thing you need most, along with humans, gadgets, instances, possibilities, and so on. It is a clearly magnetic stone with a tremendous capability to stability your mind's hemispheres. You can use this stone to help you obtain some element it is that you sincerely desire in existence.

6.24 Malachite

One of the medicinal homes of malachite crystal is its ability to adjust menstruation and cramps, ease hard artwork pain, assist with melancholy and tension, and get rid of dangerous strength from the body. It is a common tool for electricity healing, treatments, and balancing the Chakras.

6.25 Moldavite

Moldavite is notion to have extraordinary restoration residences. The metaphysical functions of moldavite's powerful vibration are speculated to open up the chakras, in particular the coronary coronary coronary heart chakra, and promote lively and spiritual recuperation whether or not or no longer or now not worn as a necklace or as a moldavite bracelet.

6.26 Moonstone

Moonstone is beneficial for exciting your female intuition and modern strain, which allows you to connect to your actual feelings. It can assist in bringing your feelings into harmony and decreasing tension. The moonstone's serene electricity stimulates innovation, restoration, and maternal safety.

6.27 Obsidian

A outstanding stone for power, protection, and grounding is obsidian. It is a root chakra stone, so it maintains you grounded within the gift and gives you a experience of internal energy and guarantee. Additionally, it protects you from terrible power and gives you the self assure to face your inner truths.

6.28 Onyx

Onyx is said to resource folks who be with the aid of sleep troubles. Stress, apathy, and neurological sicknesses are all cured with the resource of it. It lets in address eye situations like glaucoma. Onyx stone is also used to remedy blood abnormalities, bone marrow issues, and enamel troubles.

6.29 Opal

Opal has numerous makes use of. Physically, it strengthens the immune device and can be used to deal with fevers. On an emotional diploma, it may resource with harmony, enhance extremely good energy, clarity, and overcoming limitations.

6.30 Peridot

Peridot, furthermore called the stone of compassion, is concept to balance emotions and the mind to sell brilliant fitness, peaceful sleep, and concord in interpersonal relationships. In addition to inspiring eloquence and creativity, this first-class fantastic inexperienced stone additionally offers pride and appropriate cheer.

6.31 Rhodochrosite

Like the bulk of crimson gemstones, rhodochrosite vibrates to the tones of love and energy. It is frequently used to alleviate the pain of insect bites and to cope with scarring, but it additionally has great consequences at the coronary heart, strength location, and circulatory device.

6.32 Ruby

Ruby is frequently used to build internet applications. Moreover, ruby is beneficial for different programming tasks. It is often used to build servers and have a look at statistics in addition to for internet scraping and crawling.

6.33 Sapphire

The stones of statistics and peace are supposedly sapphires. They are used to deal with despair and ease stress. They are said to promote mental relaxation, meditation, and the clarity of belief required to overcome obstacles.

6.34 Selenite

This flexible stone has the power to growth your energy, calm your thoughts, and definitely rework your appearance right into a high amazing one.

6.35 Sodalite

It places a sturdy emphasis on reason, emotional harmony, instinct, and readability. The sodalite stone is used by healers trying to find perception and reality; it additionally sharpens intelligence. It has the functionality to reduce fevers and assist with insomnia.

6.36 Tanzanite

Some people take delivery of as true with that via wearing tanzanite, their cognizance can increase and their capability to understand and recollect their intuition will beautify. Some humans agree with it aids in cleaning and will increase strength. Wear it or have it close to handy for instances whilst you want a relaxing impact.

6.37 Tiger's Eye

Tiger's eye, moreover known as the stone of braveness, is useful for reinforcing your self-guarantee and energy. This stone is related to the sacrum and root chakras, therefore it aids in grounding, developing a solid foundation, and reigniting your motivation. Additionally, it without a doubt works nicely at avoiding poor electricity.

6.38 Topaz

It aids within the treatment of sleeplessness, extended memory loss, liver troubles, and jaundice. A Yellow Topaz Gemstone is also useful for liver, fever, hunger, cold and cough, and belly troubles. It treats highbrow problems, suicidal inclinations, and concerned breakdowns via calming the wearer's mind.

6.39 Tourmaline

Tourmaline aids inside the formation of a barrier spherical a person or space to hold out uninvited or risky energies. Additionally, it grounds you and aids in bringing every chakra into balance. Even extra hard impulses and destructive mind styles can be converted into more empowering energies and ideals with the useful resource of the stone.

6. Forty Zircon

Each chakra has an association with zircon. Crystal healers put it to use to cope with every physical & emotional illnesses. The blessings encompass reducing fevers, easing ache, easing stomach cramps, relieving allergic reactions, lung issues, and menstrual pain.

Part three: Improving one's lifestyles with crystals

Crystals may be used in loads of factors of your lifestyles. Crystals also can enhance your recognition and creativity if carried out in a particular manner. Additionally, crystals can useful resource inside the purification of the frame, mind, and soul. In this phase of the ebook, we are going to speak about how crystals may be beneficial in our each day lifestyles.

Chapter 7: What Crystals Can Do To Help Us In Life?

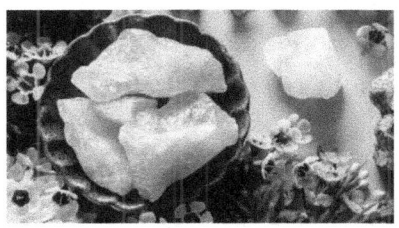

Although crystals may be implemented in a number of strategies, in trendy they offer spiritual and emotional recuperation, greater electricity and happiness, and comfort from every day strain. Additionally, they could supplement your style and are a extraordinarily-cutting-edge style announcement. The crystals with the corresponding healing features are indexed beneath.

7.1 Rose quartz, Citrine and Carnelian for positivity

One of the terrific gems for manifesting nicely emotions and strength is rose quartz. It is renowned for taking off your coronary

coronary heart chakra to sell love and peace on your surroundings. Using Rose Quartz can help you put off any intellectual limitations which can be adverse on your properly-being. Another awesome crystal for positivity is citrine. It is renowned for its capability to useful resource in elevating your easy excessive vibrations, boost your diploma of happiness, and heal emotional wounds and terrible emotions. Carnelian can beautify your temper and enjoy of well-being with the useful resource of harnessing the power of positivity.

7.2 For overcoming tension, use Rose Quartz, Green Aventurine, Sodalite, and Green Calcite

A lot of people experience tension on a private level, whether or not or not or not it is in themselves or a cherished one. Fortunately, there are numerous topics we can do to manipulate our tension. One of them is using conventional remedy options on the facet of crystal recovery houses to help us recover from our highbrow fitness troubles. For overcoming anxiety, rose quartz, green aventurine, sodalite, and inexperienced calcite may be applied.

7.Three Ruby for doing away with Addiction

The majority of crystals can offer energies which might be great for those overcoming any kind of addiction. While each person's enjoy with dependancy and restoration is precise, crystals do have some advantages that virtually every person can take gain of. The superb red stone ruby is regarded to have a great better power diploma than carnelian. Ruby can assist humans come to be greater self-aware and recognize how their moves have an effect on other people inside the international. It indeed is a first rate crystal first of all at the begin of recuperation.

7.Four The Crystals That Will Help You Manage Anger Include Green Quartz, Amazonite, Red Tiger's Eye, Labradorite and Amethyst

Crystals for anger are one of the best and most natural procedures to discover ways to manage your anger in a healthful manner. You'll experience calmer and be able to manipulate your feelings higher manner to their vibration. Although anger is a terrible emotion, it's also a regular human response to hundreds of stresses and troubles. Even even though the emotion is not unusual, harboring anger for a extended time body ought to probably restrict our increase and prevent us from experiencing abundance. The crystals an amazing manner to will let you manipulate your anger in a healthful way are green quartz, amazonite, red tiger's eye, labradorite, and amethyst.

7.Five Hematite, Rose Quartz, and Smoky Quartz can all assist one gain stability

Everyone has to address adjustments in power stages, pressure, and environmental exposures. These, but, can result in a highbrow and physical imbalance, which can make us ill. It may be time to consist of crystals for attaining stability and to decorate your famous state of being. It is feasible to balance love and intimacy the use of rose quartz. Smoky quartz is a remarkable useful aid for grounding and focusing. Your frame and thoughts may be more balanced, way to hematite.

7.6 Lapis Lazuli for Compassion

A character's honesty, compassion, and uprightness are said to be reinforced with the aid of lapis lazuli.

7.7 Decision-Making can be superior with Smoky Quartz

Smoky Quartz aids in highbrow calmness, allowing unfastened choice-making.

7.Eight Amethyst, Citrine, and Celestite for Gratitude

When seeking out to revel in gratitude, celestite is a strong gem. Celestite is useful for installing a connection to the commonplace angelic spirit. Finding thankfulness for your each day existence can be made a great deal much less tough with the help of citrine. When you want to enjoy greater appreciation or famous thankfulness to your life, amethyst is the exceptional crystal to use.

7.Nine Turquoise, Amethyst and Red Tiger's Eye for Motivation

Using crystals is one approach to growth motivation in your existence. One can experience stimulated and determined with the useful aid of the crystals. Turquoise is high-quality for enhancing motivation and self-self guarantee. Amethyst encourages better states of consciousness, which complements pressure for non secular development and a contented mind-set. Because it conjures up dedication for financial fulfillment, the crimson tiger's eye is an superb stone for industrial organisation owners.

7.10 Use Amethyst for Patience

One of the most remarkable healing crystals, amethyst is excellent for cultivating endurance. It will increase highbrow tranquilly and lessens tension and pressure.

7.Eleven Use Sapphire and Jade for Prosperity

The sapphire is regarded as a stone of abundance. Jade is also a famous stone for success and prosperity.

7.12 Stress may be managed via Jasper

The nurturing stone is jasper. It is idea to provide assist even as underneath stress.

7.Thirteen Clear quartz for reinforcing self-self perception

An remarkable stone for promoting self-self notion is plain quartz, which might also make it less complicated as a way to address your ordinary obligations. Clear quartz restores readability on your existence and serves as a steady reminder of all the top notch topics you have were given finished inside the beyond, that could assist if you've been feeling overburdened currently. It is associated with the crown chakra, which it assists in balancing and restoration.

7.14 Rose quartz, Moonstone and Ruby for Love

The stone of affection, or rose quartz, is on occasion believed to inspire be given as genuine with and love. Moonstone encourages sensations of growth and internal electricity. Ruby is idea to promote sensuality and sexuality.

Chapter 8: How To Purify Crystals

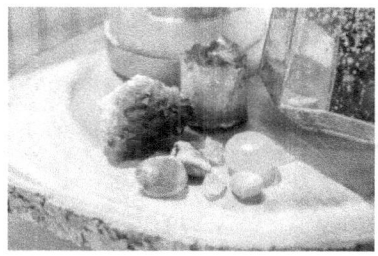

Crystals are frequently utilized by people to calm their body, mind, and spirit. Some humans think that crystals have magnetic homes and transmit the earth's inherent vibrations. Before a transaction is made, crystals often journey a exquisite distance from the deliver to the vendor. Every alternate in direction exposes stone to the energies that may not be in harmony with yours. These stones also are claimed to take in or reroute the negativity you are seeking to shed at the same time as they're used for restoration. The handiest method to move decrease lower back your crystal to its unique us of a is to often cleanse and recharge your stones. Your private experience of purpose may be revitalized by means of the use of a selected disturbing method. Here are a number of the most well-known cleaning strategies.

8.1 Running water

Any sort of awful strength held in the stone is concept to be neutralized through water and once more to the soil. You can smooth your stone below a tap or although herbal walking water from a circulate. Make fantastic your stone is very well submerged in the water, irrespective of the supply. When completed, pat it dry. Never soak your crystal in water for longer than a minute. Hard stones like quartz may be labored with this method. However, delicate or smooth stones like kyanite, selenite, and halite want to no longer be dealt with with this method.

8.2 Saltwater

Salt has been employed with the useful resource of civilizations at some point of the globe to neutralize evil vibes and purge them from their midst. You may additionally need to fill a plate with herbal saltwater from the ocean in case you take location to be in the region. If no longer, season a bowl of water with one tablespoon of rock, sea, or table salt. It's wonderful to soak the stone for anywhere from a few hours to three days. Rinse and dry it off later on. No more than forty eight hours need to be spent cleaning your stones in salt water. This machine is best for treating tough stones which include amethyst and quartz. Stones which might be porous, moderate, or include the trace metals, along side malachite, halite, selenite, calcite, lepidolite, and angelite, have to no longer be treated on this way.

8.Three Brown rice

In a ordinary and contained surroundings, this method also may be used for drawing out negativity. It works thoroughly with black tourmaline similarly to different protective stones. This can be completed thru way of concealing your stone in a dish of dry brown rice. Once you're completed with the cleaning, discard the rice as it's said to have amassed the terrible energy you are attempting to cast off. The filtering way may additionally take in to a day. In addition, this technique may be used to purify any crystal.

8. Four Natural slight

However, you may purify and recharge your stone at any time thru surely leaving it out in preference to looking for a hard and speedy time within the sun or lunar cycle. You ought to goal to get your stone lower returned inner through eleven a.M. In case you placed it out of doors at night time time. Allowing your stone to take in the solar and moonlight will allow it to do so. When sunlight hours comes, convey the stone internal, as direct daylight can harm its stop if disregarded too lengthy. Try to vicinity your stone perpendicular to the ground. Since that is possible, we are able to clean more frequently. Get rid of any people or animals that might stumble upon them. The stone need to then be quick rinsed to remove any very last dust and particles. When it is dry, provide it a short pat. It takes approximately 10-12 hours to finish this manner. Tumbled stones, in popular, can be used with this approach. Halite, celestite, and selenite are all soft stones that might be broken with the resource of manner of horrific weather, simply so they shouldn't be treated on this way. Similarly, stones with robust solar sun shades, like amethyst, ought to no longer be disregarded in direct sunlight hours.

eight.Five Sage

Sage is as an alternative regarded because of its many useful makes use of. Smudging your stone is said to dispel horrible electricity and repair its herbal electricity. To accomplish this, you may want a bowl appropriate for fireside, a lighter or fits, and both loose sage or pre-packaged sage. If you can not smudge outdoor, get near a window. Smoke and ugly vibes might be in a position to interrupt out then. Light the sage on the tip even as you're organized to begin a fire. Keep the sage in your non-dominant hand at the same time as you bypass the stone via the smoke. Allow the smoke to certainly engulf the stone for round 30 seconds. Consider smudging the stone again for a in addition 30 seconds if you have not but done it nowadays or if you have the impact that it is sticking to some element. This approach applies to any stone.

eight.6 Sound

A unmarried tone or pitch can be carried out in sound recovery to fill an area and raise its vibration to healthy the tone. Chanting, tuning fork, making a music bowls, or perhaps a ringing bell can be used to gather this. As lengthy because the song is loud sufficient to surely vibrate the stone, it does not bear in mind variety what key it's miles done in, it'll artwork. This approach is satisfactory for collectors with a number of crystals which are difficult to take report of or relocate. Any crystal can be handled the usage of this approach.

eight.7 Using a larger stone

Clearing smaller stones can be facilitated with the useful aid of using huge amethyst geodes, quartz clusters, and selenite slabs. Any of these stones can be positioned inner or on pinnacle of your stone. The imbalanced energies gift inside the resting stone are supposedly eliminated by using the vibrations of the larger stone. Any stone may be cleansed the use of this technique for a most of 24 hours.

eight.Eight Using smaller stones

Hematite, easy quartz, and carnelian also are taken into consideration to have a cleansing impact commonly. You would likely want more than this sort of stones in your hand to efficaciously put off particular stones due to the reality they will be normally smaller. The stone you want to restore must be located on top of the cleansing stones in the little bowl.

eight.Nine Breath

The cleansing strength of 1's breath is regularly left out. The first step is to hold the stone on your more potent hand. Keep your mind in your purpose at the same time as taking a few deep breaths thru your nose. Bring the stone within the course of your face and exhale fast and strongly onto it to increase its vibration. This approach works outstanding for treating smaller crystals.

eight.10 Visualization

This is stated to be the most secure approach for purifying stones. After taking a while to ground and consciousness your energy, choose out up the stone and agree with your arms are filling with a extraordinary white moderate. Visualize the stone being surrounded with the useful resource of this moderate, which you could feel getting brighter. Imagine all of the mud and dirt being washed away, revealing a purer, more useful stone. Keep doing this visualization till you word a alternate within the electricity of the stone.

Chapter 9: What Are Crystals?

What are Crystals? The time period crystal,

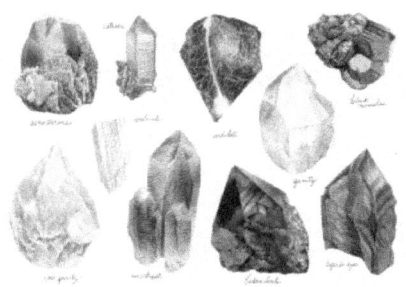

which derives from the Greek krystallos, manner a strong shape shaped by means of atoms, which is probably on the top of an ordered reticular shape and repeated an indefinite variety of instances. In exercising, the identical cells are repeated in vicinity, becoming collectively flawlessly and with none unfastened area.

I'm talking about the crystalline lattice. The lattice consequently offers an ordered form, that can lead the crystal to have described geometric shapes. The shape of a crystal is likewise very crucial in crystal treatment. We'll see why later.

The seven crystal structures are:

cubic S

S. Trigonal or rhombohedral

S. Tetragonal

S. Hexagonal

S. Monoclinic

S. Orthorhombic

S. Triclinic

In turn, they'll be grouped into 3 crystalline groups. There is the monometric (cubic s.), the dimetric (hexagonal s., tetragonal s., rhombohedral s.) and the trimetric (tricline s., monoclinic s. And the orthombic s.).

Almost all crystals are polycrystalline. In exercising, in spite of the truth that we can not frequently see it with the bare eye, they will be crafted from multiple crystals. They are microscopic structures. However, there are also monocrystals, really very unusual. The everyday is usual by way of manner of a single crystal.

How is a crystal normal?

The crystals are shaped way to a gradual solidification of a liquid or throughout the transition from aeriform to stable of a fuel. It must no longer undergo the liquid one. The developments assumed by way of the crystal depend, as an example, at the price with which it solidifies and what the conditions are.

These rocks can be magmatic (primary formation), i.E. Born from the solidification of magmas. They may be sedimentary (secondary formation), i.E. From the buildup of sediments and which arise in maximum times from the erosion of pre-present rocks. Finally they will be metamorphic (tertiary formation), they arrive from the transformation of other rocks.

How to apply crystals

Taken from a communicate that clearly befell:

"The amethyst calms me and the crimson jasper gives me energy, proper?"

"... It depends, perhaps it is probably higher in case you understood greater deeply the origins of the scenario you're experiencing before counting on any form of remedy ..."

"But I've observe that an amethyst pendant is a wonderful remedy for my tension! It isn't so?"

"... It depends..."

Yes, it's far based upon! The use of crystals in holistic practices has (regularly) emerge as a few difficulty that carefully resembles the horoscopes which might be study in newspapers.

The opportunity that the universe, and consequently the celebrities, could have interplay with human affairs is an ancient question, however that a brief paragraph of some lines can be appropriate for truely anyone born under that specific signal is a very constructive forecast!

Unfortunately, we often witness a similar situation for crystal magic. In this financial ruin we are going to dispel the maximum common myths on the assignment and discover the manner to use crystals effectively in keeping with their homes and our non-public state of affairs.

Why do crystals paintings?

We have already investigated the bodily reasons inside the back of the interactions with crystals and it's time to discover a little deeper the query.

We will keep in thoughts that the precept elements that function their competencies to minerals are their symbolic fee (that might rely upon historical, cultural and personal elements) and their intrinsic homes. Now we're capable of try to find out this second detail, that would emerge as vital for an effective and conscious use of crystals.

Physical and energetic homes of crystals

From this point of view, the factors that most have an impact at the talents of a mineral (i.E. Its morphogenesis) are two:

its bodily composition;

the perception we have were given of it.

These peculiarities make the crystals an entire lot extra understandable and everyday with numerous ancient disciplines, which encompass yoga, traditional Chinese medicinal drug, Ayurveda, Tantrism and others.

Let's begin with the number one of the traits.

Physical composition

The morphogenesis of a mineral is the end result of the geological techniques that generated it. Let's undergo in mind one of the maximum charming and exceptional minerals, rock crystal. This, better defined as hyaline quartz, belongs to the mineral institution of oxides and in particular of quartz, among which it stands proud for its specific transparency, actually much like glass.

Quartz is a not unusual detail of acidic intrusive igneous rocks (together with granite as an instance), but is likewise located abundantly in sedimentary ones (collectively with sandstone).

From the element of view of physical composition, quartzes have a trigonal crystalline shape, inclusive of multiple tetrahedra joined collectively thru the four vertices, forming spirals orientated to the right or left. Its shape (habitus) is a hexagonal prism with the faces of two rhombohedra at the pinnacle prepared to form a hexagonal-based bi-pyramid.

Finally, hyaline quartz appears as a crystal proper now recognizable for the feel of purity it is able to transmit, moreover way to its singular transparency. Once accumulated by way of way of the exhibitor, we also can be capable of appreciate its weight, freshness and smoothness, perceiving a incredible present day balance.

Power

In mild of what we've got just stated, every of these factors will make a contribution to giving the rock crystal its valuable houses.

Color, geological origins and physical composition will translate proper right right into a vibratory float of complicated and deeply articulated harmonies.

To summarize, we're confronted with a stone that can be of every lava and sedimentary beginning, consequently near each yang (fireplace) and yin (water) elements. It has a pyramidal habitus with a triangular base, one of the maximum strong shapes in nature however additionally that awesome represents the connection between earth and sky. To the touch it's miles bloodless and really smooth, but it is able to amaze with the subtlety of its profiles, sharp but on the equal time fragile.

Perception

To recognize the viable results on someone, however, each of its tendencies must be associated with the right situation of the latter, located, as an example, through one or more of the disciplines stated. An Ayurvedic practitioner - even as now not the use of these tool inside the number one - can also moreover discover it beneficial to apply the homes of rock crystal to intervene on one or more of the fundamental energies gift within the man or woman (ether, air, fireplace, water and earth).

Similarly, a practitioner of conventional Chinese treatment need to depend upon the male and lady components to restore balance to the situation's qi electricity.

A gourmand of yoga or tantrism may be led to use hyaline quartz to behave on one or more electricity centers, exploiting as an instance the electricity vibrations inside the seen spectrum, that is the colour.

To this already glaring complexity is delivered the reality that minerals have a restrained fashion of movement in place. This way that their place also can be decisive for the effectiveness of the movement!

Indeed, we're capable to mention that placing the right crystal within the incorrect vicinity no longer amazing renders it ineffective, but potentially transforms it right right into a purpose of undesirable, if now not awful, consequences.

This attention is legitimate whether or not or now not one uses movements on the doshas (essential energy individual for Ayurveda), whether or not one acts on the meridians (electricity channels of conventional Chinese remedy) and, subsequently, that one intends to interfere on the functioning of the chakras (electricity facilities Hinduism).

Chapter 10: How To Apply Crystals The Right Manner: Strength And Notion

We now begin to understand why we from time to time pay interest, as an instance, to bring that unique crystal to one aspect instead of each other in the body. This indication, but, should most effective be understood as a tremendous tenet. In truth, if every crystal could have one or more places wherein it manifests a particular famous concord, there can be no point in itself "wrong" to place it. Wrong - that is, not desired - there can excellent be the effect it produces!

To deliver an example, setting a black tourmaline at the peak of the better chakras is typically now not encouraged, however there can be situations wherein that is the maximum appropriate intervention for the specific scenario. Likewise, pink jasper is frequently associated with the primary or second chakra however, in nice situations, it could produce undesirable consequences. However, those aren't results opposite to expectancies, as the ones need to be based totally on entire know-how of the stone used, similarly to at the understanding of the proper case to which it's far to be implemented.

For this cause, it want to commonly be considered that the purpose to be looked for a person's actual nicely-being is to sell their lively and realistic homeostasis. This is the circumstance of most viable stability, in which power flows without difficulty, growing an regular concord a number of the material and immaterial dimensions of the individual.

For this reason, excessive attention is wanted within the use of crystal magic. The use of a mineral in a unmarried trouble of the body in preference to every other will produce the equal energetic effect this is right to it, however the sensible outcomes - that is, the feedback experienced with the aid of the individual - may be substantially one in every of a type relying on their unique situations.

In different words, if we're considering the opportunity of the usage of a few crystal magic treatments lightly because of the fact a lot "it doesn't harm", probable it is higher that we desist from this goal. With these premises the quality end result we are able to aspire to, in fact, might be their ineffectiveness, with out prejudice to the feasible placebo impact.

If, however, we preferred to take whole benefit of the assist of the representatives of the mineral international - very effective allies and every now and then even accomplices - then we learn how to use them as efficaciously as possible, combining this preliminary understanding with an facts of our conditions. Knowing ourselves and our energies is critical as a way to apply the crystals correctly and make the most of their residences.

Finally, a concluding mirrored image on crystal magic in giant. In attention of its holistic nature, of its essential complementarity to actual medication and, specifically, of the intrinsic empirical price of the notions deriving from it, it might be best to are trying to find advice from it with the time period of crystal practice, consequently following the course already marked thru particular disciplines in the modern day beyond.

The "full" and "empty" of remember range

The atomic tool, in the collective creativeness, is a difficult and fast of microscopic solar systems wherein the nucleus represents the sun, at the same time because the electrons end up the planets that revolve spherical it.

However, the remark of the functioning of atoms quickly observed that electrons did now not take a look at conventional orbits which include Newton's predefined ones for celestial bodies. Their trajectory appeared as an alternative unpredictable, but the distance that the electrons maintained from the nucleus.

Unable to calculate their orbits, the researchers then centered their interest on the gap the various nucleus and electrons.

But how some distance is an electron from the nucleus? Since those measures are so small as to be difficult to understand, it's miles profitable to make an example with more commonly used objects.

If we may additionally want to expand an atomic nucleus to the size of an apple we would have to move about 1 km away to satisfy the primary electron. Imagining an atom as easy as hydrogen in those dimensions, we might find out that it's miles composed of our apple (the nucleus) and, approximately a kilometer away, a unmarried electron. It is a big vicinity occupied thru little or no don't forget. The ratio among complete and empty is in truth same to one millionth of a millionth!

Therefore remember wide variety is in most cases "empty". It need to not be unexpected that this interest leaves our kids astonished at the same time as they're new to physics. In fact, it took a long term to recognize the manner it have grow to be feasible that two portions of matter repelled every other thru getting into contact, as opposed to merging on the atomic stage, due to the fact the enormity of empty area may additionally additionally lead us to anticipate.

The solution end up placed with the resource of Max Plank with a discovery that, in 1918, earned him the Nobel Prize in physics and which can be summarized by means of the usage of the usage of his famous declaration:

"Matter does no longer exist, the whole lot is vibration!"

A certainly enlightened intuition.

From atoms to thread idea

Wanting to simplify beyond degree, the solidity of atoms is because of electromagnetic forces - and the "orbits" of electrons are in reality actual electromagnetic fields.

We consider a place as the feel of a cloth in which each unmarried filament suggests a specific interaction. The threads are so dense that it now not makes enjoy to do not forget them in my opinion, but the cloth as a whole want to be considered. In our case, that vicinity placed approximately one kilometer from the apple is the electromagnetic discipline of our hydrogen atom.

But to recognize how our loved crystals can engage with the rest of depend - which makes up everything, even our our our bodies - we want to increase the magnification of our imaginary microscope a hint in addition and have a look at don't forget in its maximum intimate nature, past below atoms. We communicate exactly of sub-atomic physics to define the take a look at of the smallest particles of atoms.

In reality, we have already encountered 3 of them, protons, neutrons and electrons, however the zoo of primary particles is an entire lot more nourished and continuously seems organized to welcome new animals, every with its very personal peculiarities and useful for the functioning of depend extensive variety and of the universe (or as a substitute, to our know-how of it).

In truth, we talk of quarks, leptons, hadrons and the listing in no manner appears to forestall, swelling its ranks every time it is important to find out the individual accountable for some effect or new launch.

Someone then asked himself a question: what if there was something more radical to offer an explanation for the functioning of count number in a definitive, elegant manner and without resorting to such numerous debris?

The concept of string principle have become born from the hypothesis that some thing even smaller and extra elusive want to exist, however capable of defining all possible particles.

Chapter 11: The Power Strings And The Concept Of Vibration

Strings are entities without rely and composed remarkable of vibrating energy. The variability in their form and vibration is in a position to distinguish every type of debris, consequently, additionally of rely.

Fifty years after Plank's Nobel Prize, the Italian Gabriele Veneziano sensed the existence of strings, however it took some other two years for a few physicists to virtually increase the concept. In 1974, Schwarz and Sherk thru way of enhancing the vibration modes of the strings acquired a particle equal to 2, or the graviton.

After a few different 10 years, Green and Schwarz defined nearly all of the phenomena of interaction of depend via strings, definitively attracting the eye of the scientific network and redefining, in all likelihood as quickly as and for all, the very concept we have were given of depend: no more corpuscles. Mins that stir inside the air, but instead a diffuse symphony of vibrations.

Plank himself, close to his earthly quit, wrote

"Having dedicated my whole lifestyles to the most rational technological understanding viable, the have a study of be counted, I can assist you to realise at least this about my studies at the atom: rely as such does no longer exist! All depend exists quality through specific function of a stress that makes the debris vibrate and continues this tiny sun device of the atom. We can count on under this force, the life of an 'Intelligent and aware Spirit'. This Spirit is the reason for all remember quantity. "

After no a fantastic deal a whole lot less than four thousand years, Western physics has positioned traces of the Hindu ether. Akasha is in truth the time period to signify the simple and primary essence of all topics within the cloth worldwide, whose intrinsic feature, like region - Aristotelian non-being - turn out to be to make all subjects exist inside it. Akasha is the quintessence, the substratum of Shabda, that is, of sound, the important vibration.

The vibration of the crystals

So, returning to crystal magic, the whole lot vibrates. All depend is itself a form of very complex vibration.

Like our frame, or rather the atoms that make up the molecules that all and sundry together call "frame", the crystals additionally vibrate. When an oscillating device (something that vibrates) is subjected to periodic stresses with frequencies identical to the oscillation of the tool itself, the phenomenon called "resonance" takes vicinity.

The most effective instance to breed is that of a couple of tuning forks: the oscillations produced through the percussion of a tuning fork prompt an equal tuning fork to vibrate and, therefore, to reproduce the same frequency. This phenomenon has a vital cost in our reasoning due to the truth, further to being the purpose why we do now not sink into nothing on the equal time as we lean on a chair, it moreover explains how interaction with crystals can be completed.

Like a few different "element" inside the universe, rocks and crystals vibrate and every crystal does so at unique frequencies. These can, like some one-of-a-kind vibration, create resonant effects with some thing else, which incorporates us.

The resonance between the human body and the crystals

Obviously, the mechanism is a piece more complex than tuning the radio to the frequencies of our favourite broadcaster.

As with acupuncture, Ayurveda and conventional Chinese medicine, for millennia sensible experimentation has modified scientific demonstration. When Western medical doctors went looking for the energy meridians, so powerful in the remedy of pain, they located not anything, deducing that the ones truly did not exist. The same goes for the chakras. In reality, any practitioner of Chinese medication spoke back that they could not find out them, really because of the truth they had been not "fabric", but represented electricity resonance channels, flows in which strength created resonance outcomes.

Minerals (or maybe more so crystals) art work in the equal way. Their frequency - determined through their atomic shape - can create a resonance impact with some factors of our body. And, inside the absence of clinical evidence, crystal magic can rent the experience obtained over the millennia via guys of all latitudes.

In truth, there is no region in the global in which a few stones had been no longer recognized with a selected electricity. However, if those abilities can not trade over time, for the motive that they rely upon the deep interaction among fabric and energetic elements, what has certainly modified is us.

The golden rule to use of crystals

In this regard, we're able to say that there are three essential rules that allow us to make the exceptional use of crystals:

Clean (each bodily and etherically), a superb way to put off each dirt from the ground of the stone, and stagnant or congested energies; cleansing is completed with Marseille cleansing soap (ideally herbal) and cold water; in this regard it is ideal to bear in mind that it isn't possible to purify the stones in boiling water, otherwise the stone may want to break or lose its luster;

Charge (under the solar's rays or the crescent or entire moon) so that it will supply renewed and smooth power to the crystal; about ninety% of the crystals ought to be uncovered to the overall moon, however there are a few exceptions (as in the case, as an example, of Smoky Quartz or Carnelian);

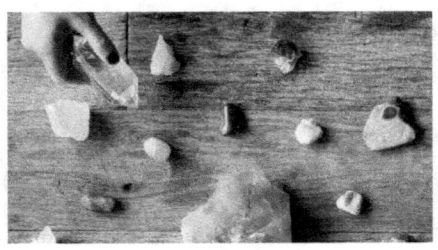

Program, in case you want to give unique instructions and a specific challenge to our stone; because of this it's miles crucial to have a mind loose from any troubles, focusing each at the gestures and on the motive with which we need to software the crystal.

Best crystals for beginners

In this segment I go away you the crystals that I recall critical for any beginner. They are high-quality for buying started out out inside the magic of minerals and you ought to now not have a brilliant deal trouble getting them at a first rate charge.

Rose quartz (pink)

If there may be a mineral which you need to have on your room, it's miles rose quartz. It is a mineral that attracts self-love, love for a companion and compassion. Rose quartz is capable of converting the environment and lowering anger in an trouble, calming down the spirits and welcoming talk. It furthermore invitations friendship and reconciliation.

Tourmaline (black)

As I definitely have commented, black stones are typically focused on protection. Black tourmaline is one of the minerals with the maximum protective energy. It is so powerful that it can block horrible energies directed at you and turn them into best electricity. It additionally has the capability to repel electromagnetic waves from electric domestic gadget, so it's miles encouraged to have a tourmaline bracelet or pendant if you artwork with computer structures or digital gadgets. You can location black tourmaline close to your tv and laptop at domestic. This mineral may even help you focus and assume certainly.

Tiger eye (orange)

Another stone that works as a protector is the tiger's eye, the attention that is privy to everything. If you want to shield your private home, place some tiger's eye stones at the entrance of your home and they will be chargeable for the usage of away terrible power and horrible intentions from feasible intruders. This mineral moreover complements optimism and balance in existence. If you're starting a venture, the tiger's eye will assist you focus, be more innovative and placed the whole thing in order.

Clear quartz (white)

Surely you've got got got ever visible clear quartz crystals. They are very commonplace with reference to meditating and performing spells and requests. This form of crystals incorporates silica, a completely commonplace mineral inside the composition of the earth's crust and which lets in a smooth and direct connection with the earth. Its apparent nature lets in to accumulate clarity and is proper for leaving your mind smooth, something difficult if you are new to meditation. Clear quartz may also even assist you remove physical blockages and allow strength to go together with the float more effortlessly.

Amethyst (crimson)

One of the dream crystals par excellence is amethyst. Placed subsequent to the bed or beneath the pillow it facilitates to enhance intuition and prophetic goals if the witch is vulnerable to them. If you've got got quite a few nightmares, attempt putting an amethyst stone on your nightstand. The purpose is to smooth and loosen up your thoughts before slumbering and assist you keep away from having terrible desires. If nightmares are a normal hassle for you, don't forget to purify and recharge your amethyst stones frequently, as the ones will collect quite some wasted power and negativity. Amethyst is likewise an wonderful mineral to use in meditation, because it helps channel the spirit towards concord and calm.

Aventurine (green)

If you are trying to attraction to fortune and coins, bear in mind to hold an aventurine stone on your handbag or purse. It will now not have a mind-blowing and immediate effect however, in case you are insightful and attentive, you'll be aware how it is a good deal less hard in case you want to keep and get cash given which you have the aventurine for your bag. It is likewise an outstanding enchantment for exams or task interviews. You can gift an aventurine stone to a loved one earlier than an essential event. Remember to rate the crystal in advance than an vital event and reputation your triumphing need through doing so. If you preserve studying you can find out the commands to recharge your minerals

Sodalite (blue)

This is one in every of my favored crystals. When it entails taking a comforting and enjoyable bathtub, placing numerous sodalite stones in the bath will assist lessen collected anxiety and stress. Sodalite is a mineral this is used to address each the thoughts and the frame. This stone will will let you to recharge your batteries within the course of the night time time, to acquire a deep calm and to rest properly, as a give up end result it is also used inside the bed room.

Heliotrope or bloodstone (purple)

Bloodstone is a in fact mysterious mineral, black, dark inexperienced, and crimson in coloration. It is known as the stone of fitness and serves to deal with health problems with the resource of using placing the stone at the vicinity that has the ailment. For instance, in case your nose bleeds, you can region a blood stone at the decrease again of your neck and it's going to forestall the drift, as it has a unique effect at the bloodstream.

Chapter 12: Benefits Of Crystal Treatment

The houses of stones and crystals had been exploited for masses of years and a number of the maximum historic civilizations, along side Egyptians and Maya specifically, used crystals in the path of ceremonies, to divine the future, as a lucky attraction and for the treatment of unique ailments.

Although the effectiveness of crystal treatment isn't scientifically examined and its results are attributed to the placebo effect, although nowadays stones and crystals are utilized by many individuals who recognize their benefits on a highbrow, religious, emotional and physical level.

The homes of minerals are especially exploited for:

Rebalance energies;

bring nicely-being in case of strain, tension, agitation and different emotional states that could motive or worsen physical illnesses.

The stones, moving into resonance with people who use them, deliver serenity and assist relieve muscle tension, pain, digestive troubles, insomnia and different strain-related symptoms.

There are super forms of crystals which are prominent with the useful resource of color and homes, as they paintings on particular Chakras:

For instance, the emerald is normally endorsed to convey clarity to thoughts;

topaz favors optimism;

rose quartz lets in to do away with issues.

In addition to differing in colour, form and homes and further to being related to a Chakra, every crystal is associated with an detail and a zodiac sign.

Getting started out with crystals: for beginners!

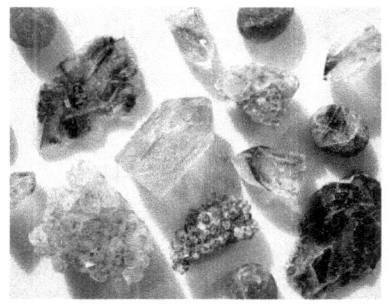

Magic crystals and minerals have always been a way of channeling energies and reinforcing intentions. There are crystals that appeal to fortune, others that balance the surroundings, others that sell particular health ... That is why it is so important that a amateur has her first magic crystals as rapid as possible, to discover ways to use them and to song in to them.

It is likewise essential which you keep in thoughts that the crystals are a complement to the set of each day magic and no longer decisive items to be able to alternate your life from in some unspecified time in the future to the subsequent. They are not miracles, they will be accomplices of your journey and you need to harmonize.

With this segment you will test the which means of severa crystals and minerals and, most importantly, a manner to use them for your every day lifestyles. Here I supply an cause in the back of a way to apply the crystals and the way to easy and rate them. And, of route, I advocate the eight high-quality magic crystals to get you commenced, smooth to get and espresso-fee.

eight is a magic extensive range in China, it symbolizes splendid fortune. For this reason, on the 8th of the 8th month of 2008, at 8 pm, eight minutes and eight seconds, the Olympic Games have been inaugurated in China. In this way, achievement would accompany all the celebrations that were to return lower lower back.

However, the range eight moreover has a special and magical this means that that has transcended in time. The eight symbolizes infinity, the start and the stop associated. And that is why I without a doubt have selected this amount to offer the eight magic crystals a good way to accompany you all through your existence, from the begin of your witch path to the end.

It is a non-public choice. In the give up, you may choose to have extra than eight crystals, or five of the most crucial are enough. It all is based upon to your magical path, your fortunate range or the range that has the greatest which means that on your life.

The importance of colors

Although every crystal or mineral has its non-public magical essence, its which means that and its usefulness, initially, you may classify minerals and stones via their shades. This will help you rapid end up aware about them and use them to your ordinary existence. Of path, maintain in thoughts that that is a type in ultra-modern terms.

Yellow electricity, success, development, pride water, recovery, communique, concept clarity, purity, communication magic, goals, clairvoyance, spirituality.

Black safety, defend sexuality, fertility, stability, creativity, energy ardour, love, power self-love, friendship, restoration, romance, consensus.

Green money, abundance, nature.

There are minerals that, even though their shade shows, for instance, energy, ought to have a deeper and extra complete which means that. So I normally suggest that, when you have time, look at a piece greater in every of your crystals.

crystal remedy

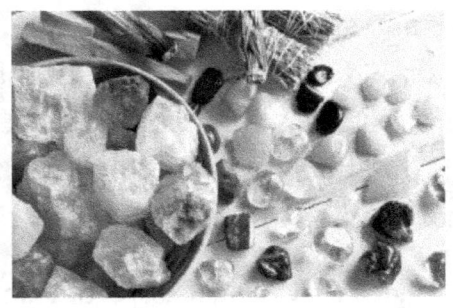

Crystal remedy is an historic alternative treatment that uses crystals, stones and minerals in case you want to reap and hold a rustic of psycho-physical well-being.

Crystal treatment is based totally on an assumption common to different holistic disciplines and traditional drug treatments in line with which there is an strength imbalance behind a bodily illness or emotional ache.

In truth, man may be capable of absorb energies thru the Chakras, gateways to the important strength glide of the frame, and to transform them. If the body absorbs terrible energies or if imbalances are created, health issues upward thrust up.

According to crystal treatment, every stone is able to protect in opposition to horrible or risky energies, emanate purifying energies and regulate the body's strength stability, restoring bodily and intellectual well-being. Often the removal of energy blockages thru crystals is supported via manner of other practices which includes aromatherapy and Reiki.

Despite not having clinical proof, the recovery thoughts of crystal therapy, additionally shared by using manner of using Yoga, Acupuncture and Ayurveda, are not in contradiction with present day clinical studies.

Chapter 13: Creating The Best Crystals Grid

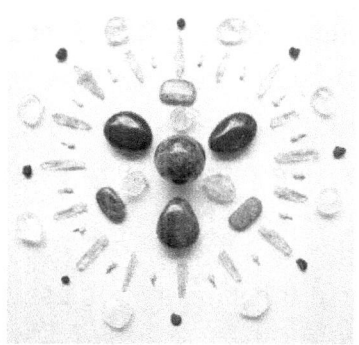

The Crystal Grids are a technology for attracting energy and vibrations in order that preferred manifestations are less complicated to accumulate with readability and deep this means that.

1. Define a purpose or reason that you want to carry out along with your grid.

Be unique. Your mind must be very smooth about what you want.

Choose one purpose at a time and focus on it.

Ideally it may be suitable to create your grid within the section of a cutting-edge-day moon, which represents new beginnings.

Want to supply extra abundance into your lifestyles? Do you need to achieve your fitness desires? Need to reinforce your creativity? Are you seeking out assist to sleep higher at night?

The opportunities are endless; you may create a grid of crystals to show up any purpose.

2. Find a steady vicinity to installation your grid wherein it could not be disturbed.

Clean your devoted crystal grid area. Some cleansing techniques encompass burning sage, or palo santo, and setting bowls of sea salt and crystal druses across the room.

Flowers, incense, music, candles may be used to feature environment in your sacred space.

Place the grid in the appropriate place of the residence in which it is not in all likelihood to be touched or disturbed (which includes thru youngsters or pets).

You can also create your grid on a tray or board so it can be moved spherical if wanted.

three. Choose the form of sacred geometry that can help you gain your cause.

Choose the form suitable on your aim to set up the crystals that you could choose out moreover primarily based on the gap you have were given to be had.

There are many grid designs based mostly on sacred geometry. Use a smooth geometric form within the starting. Grids do now not need to be complex to paintings properly.

It is also feasible to create grids with out a hard and fast geometry and revel in intuitively interested in specific patterns on the way to paintings and balance power in just the right manner to perform your aim.

4. Choose crystals and stones which can be aligned collectively along with your purpose.

If you are seeking to create an abundance grid, you may bear in mind running with crystals that could bring abundance, which includes Aventurine, Citrine, Pyrite.

If, as a substitute, you are developing a health and wellness grid, you can use blue and red crystals as recuperation stones together with Fluorite, Sodalite, Angelite, and so forth.

There aren't any proper and wrong stones to apply. Choose individuals who hobby you. Trust your instinct.

five. Make superb your crystals are smooth and charged.

You can clean them with any method you need. Then rate your crystals via preserving them among your hands and interest on the strength or impact you need to get out of your crystal, which include protection or abundance.

The maximum vital detail about a grid is the purpose used even as putting it up. Hold every single crystal on your hand and consciousness on what you want. Simply preserve it on your palms using specific keywords like "expand," "abundance," or "love."

You also can maintain the crystals all collectively in your palms and visualize what you are trying to take location to your lifestyles. For instance, in case you are looking for your ideal courting, recollect living it and feeling the pleasure related to your desire as though it had been already fulfilled with the useful resource of shielding the crystals in your hands.

6. Write your aim on a chunk of paper.

Then fold the written purpose and set it aside or you could vicinity it in the center of your grid or in near proximity.

When writing your reason, try and be as precise as feasible.

7. Arrange your crystals.

A vital grid includes 4, 5, 6 or 7 or extra stones; commonly one in the center and the relaxation spherical it located on a sheet with the chosen (sacred) geometry determine.

Place every stone (together with your purpose loaded) right right into a geometric association (or intuitive form or format), ensuring to look at the strains of the geometry of the shape.

Proper alignment is needed for correct strength go with the float.

You can region your intention written below the stone inside the center of your crystal grid.

eight. Activate the grid made with a brief thanksgiving prayer..

To spark off, recharge and empower your grid, you could use a rock crystal or selenite quartz wand or you may energize your grid with gadget or some thing feels proper and works great for you. Some use Buddhist mantras to fee the grids.

An possibility technique of activating the grid is to "draw" 3 circles clockwise, along with your wand, throughout the grid (in case your motive is to function strength to the state of affairs) or 3 circles counterclockwise around the grid (if your purpose is to cast off energy from the state of affairs).

9. Grid safety.

Always don't forget to easy the stones frequently with the aid of passing them through a few incense which include sage or palo santo as, as an example, at the same time as you are developing the grid.

You need to set apart a bit time each day (on the identical time as low as a couple of minutes) to connect with your grid power and reason.

You may additionally select out to do that via meditating and this will make your grid an area of private electricity or self-recuperation and assist you boom your grid energy (through your aware use of it).

If your grid is disturbed (kids, cats, and so forth) and crystals are touched and moved out of alignment, the grid will need to be reactivated. Also, in case you add stones to the grid or flow stones away, the grid will have to be reactivated.

10. Remove the grid

When you're completed using the grid, you can bypass decrease lower back the stones to the earth as it's far their womb, in which they arrive from.

The nice and handiest strength grid is one created following your heart and intuition.

Make sure your goals are smooth, great, and correct-oriented. There isn't always any "proper or wrong" way to do that.

Chapter 14: History Of Crystal Healing

The Use of Crystals in Ancient Cultures

The use of crystals in restoration and non secular practices dates lower returned loads of years, with evidence in their use determined in historic cultures at some stage in the globe. From the Egyptians and Greeks to the Native Americans and Chinese, crystals had been reputable for their effective energy and recovery houses.

The Egyptians have been appeared for their advanced information of astrology, alchemy, and non secular practices. They believed that crystals held effective power and used them in an entire lot of methods. For instance, they used lapis lazuli to symbolize the sky and turquoise to symbolize the earth. They extensively utilized crystals in earrings, amulets, and talismans for protection and healing. The Egyptians believed that crystals had the capability to expand energy, and could use them in their restoration practices to beautify the body's natural recuperation competencies.

Similarly, the Greeks believed that crystals were normal from the tears of the gods and that they held powerful recuperation electricity. They used crystals in their treatment and recovery practices, and masses in their clinical remedies included using crystals. For example, they could use hematite to save you bleeding and amethyst to therapy drunkenness. They additionally believed that sure crystals had the energy to keep off evil spirits and defend in competition to bad electricity.

The Native Americans have a deep reverence for the natural worldwide and believed that the whole thing in nature had a spirit and strength. They used crystals of their remedy and recuperation practices and believed that they will help to balance the frame's power and promote restoration. They substantially carried out crystals of their spiritual ceremonies and believed that they'll assist to connect them to the spirit worldwide. For instance, the Apache tribe used turquoise in their remedy baggage for protection and healing, at the same time as the Navajo used crystals in their sand paintings for religious recuperation.

The Chinese have an extended facts of the use of crystals of their medicinal drug and healing practices. They believed that crystals held effective strength and that they may assist to stability the body's power and promote recuperation. They significantly implemented crystals in their non secular practices and believed that they will assist to connect them to the divine. For instance, they could use jade to represent the coronary heart and amethyst to symbolize the zero.33 eye chakra. They additionally believed that one of a kind crystals had one-of-a-type recuperation houses and might use them as a result.

Crystals were utilized in healing and spiritual practices in lots of precise cultures as nicely.

The Aztecs used obsidian for protection and the Mayans used jade for healing. The ancient Persians used agate for healing and the Romans used amethyst for safety. The Vikings used amber for protection and the Celts used quartz for divination.

The use of crystals in recovery and non secular practices is a acquainted practice that transcends time and subculture. Crystals have been applied in hundreds of ways, from jewelry and amulets to remedy and religious practices. Their use remains a powerful device for selling balance, concord, and internal peace.

The Pioneers of Modern Crystal Healing

The use of crystals for restoration has skilled a resurgence in recognition in contemporary years, with many humans searching out alternative varieties of healing and properly being. While using crystals in restoration and non secular practices dates again hundreds of years, there were several pioneers in modern crystal recovery who've helped to supply this historical practice to a much broader target market.

One of the most famous pioneers of current-day crystal recuperation is Marcel Vogel. Vogel changed into a research scientist who labored for IBM within the 1950s and Nineteen Sixties. He become inquisitive about the residences of quartz crystals and commenced experimenting with them in his spare time. Vogel determined that he must use a completely unique decreasing technique to beautify the electricity of the crystal, and he went on to boom a tool of crystal recovery that he referred to as "Vogel Crystals." Vogel believed that those crystals is probably used to extend the electricity of the human body and sell healing.

Another pioneer of current-day crystal recovery is Katrina Raphaell. Raphaell is an creator and crystal healer who has written numerous books at the undertaking, together with "The Crystalline Transmission" and "Crystal Enlightenment." She has advanced a device of crystal restoration that consists of using particular crystals and their corresponding chakras. Raphaell believes that crystals can be used to stability and harmonize the frame's electricity, and she or he or he has advanced a series of strategies that can be used to sell restoration and properly-being.

Judy Hall is every different well-known pioneer of contemporary crystal restoration. Hall is an writer and crystal healer who has written severa books on the state of affairs, together with "The Crystal Bible" and "The Encyclopedia of Crystals." She has developed a gadget of crystal recuperation that includes the usage of precise crystals and their corresponding houses. Hall believes that crystals can be used to enhance the body's herbal recovery abilities and sell religious growth.

Melody is a few one-of-a-kind influential decide in cutting-edge crystal recovery. Melody is an writer and crystal healer who has written several books on the issue, along side "Love Is In The Earth" and "The Master Book of Healing Crystals." She has advanced a system of crystal restoration that consists of the usage of unique crystals and their corresponding houses. Melody believes that crystals can be used to heal the frame, thoughts, and spirit, and they may be used to attach us to the divine.

Naisha Ahsian is also a exceptional figure in contemporary crystal recovery. Ahsian is an author and crystal healer who has written numerous books on the assignment, consisting of "The Book of Stones" and "Crystal Resonance." She has superior a machine of crystal recuperation that carries the usage of unique crystals and their corresponding homes. Ahsian believes that crystals may be used to align the body's energy with that of the earth and the universe, and they will be used to sell non secular boom and transformation.

The pioneers of current crystal healing have helped to deliver this historical workout to a miles broader purpose market. These people have advanced structures of crystal recuperation that include the use of precise crystals and their corresponding houses. They receive as proper with that crystals may be used to balance and harmonize the frame's energy, decorate the body's natural recovery abilties, and sell religious growth and transformation. The work of these pioneers has helped to installation crystal restoration as a legitimate shape of opportunity restoration and well-being.

The Science Behind Crystal Healing

Crystal recuperation is a workout that has been used for loads of years, but its effectiveness and the underlying mechanisms were a topic of discussion within the scientific community. Some humans acquire as proper with that crystals have restoration houses due to their specific molecular shape and electromagnetic houses, even as others argue that the benefits of crystal recovery are due to the placebo impact. In cutting-edge years, clinical studies were finished to research the technology within the back of crystal healing.

One of the maximum crucial additives of crystal recuperation is the unique molecular structure of crystals. Crystals are made from atoms that are organized in a particular pattern. This molecular shape gives crystals precise homes, which includes their functionality to conduct strength. Some crystals are capable of behavior electric power, at the same time as others are capable of conduct warmth electricity. This specific molecular form is one of the reasons why crystals are believed to have healing homes.

Another important detail of crystal restoration s the electromagnetic homes of crystals. Crystals have an electromagnetic place that interacts with the electromagnetic difficulty of the human frame. This interplay is idea to help stability the strength of the frame and promote restoration. Some crystals, which incorporates quartz, are able to emit a regular electromagnetic discipline, which is assumed to enhance their restoration houses.

Scientific research have tested that crystals will have a measurable effect at the human frame. One have a look at completed in 2001 positioned that the electromagnetic issue of a quartz crystal had a relaxing effect at the brain. Another take a look at performed in 2018 discovered that wearing a necklace made from amethyst had a effective impact on the mood and strength degrees of members.

www.ingramcontent.com/pod-product-compliance
Lightning Source LLC
Chambersburg PA
CBHW071440080526
44587CB00014B/1932